Department of Veterans Affairs
Health Services Research & Development Service | Evidence-based Synthesis Program

Mobile Applications and Internet-based Approaches for Supporting Non-professional Caregivers: A Systematic Review

November 2012

Prepared for:
Department of Veterans Affairs
Veterans Health Administration
Quality Enhancement Research Initiative
Health Services Research & Development Service
Washington, DC 20420

Prepared by:
Evidence-based Synthesis Program (ESP) Center
Portland VA Medical Center
Portland, OR
Devan Kansagara, M.D., M.C.R., Director

Investigators:
Principal Investigator:
Edward A. Dyer, M.D.

Co-Investigators:
Devan Kansagara, M.D., M.C.R.
D. Keith McInnes, Sc.D., M.Sc.
Michele Freeman, M.P.H.
Susan Woods, M.D., M.P.H.

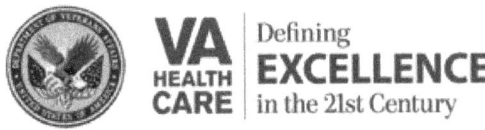

PREFACE

Quality Enhancement Research Initiative's (QUERI) Evidence-based Synthesis Program (ESP) was established to provide timely and accurate syntheses of targeted healthcare topics of particular importance to Veterans Affairs (VA) managers and policymakers, as they work to improve the health and healthcare of Veterans. The ESP disseminates these reports throughout VA.

QUERI provides funding for four ESP Centers and each Center has an active VA affiliation. The ESP Centers generate evidence syntheses on important clinical practice topics, and these reports help:
- develop clinical policies informed by evidence,
- guide the implementation of effective services to improve patient outcomes and to support VA clinical practice guidelines and performance measures, and
- set the direction for future research to address gaps in clinical knowledge.

In 2009, the ESP Coordinating Center was created to expand the capacity of QUERI Central Office and the four ESP sites by developing and maintaining program processes. In addition, the Center established a Steering Committee comprised of QUERI field-based investigators, VA Patient Care Services, Office of Quality and Performance, and Veterans Integrated Service Networks (VISN) Clinical Management Officers. The Steering Committee provides program oversight, guides strategic planning, coordinates dissemination activities, and develops collaborations with VA leadership to identify new ESP topics of importance to Veterans and the VA healthcare system.

Comments on this evidence report are welcome and can be sent to Nicole Floyd, ESP Coordinating Center Program Manager, at nicole.floyd@va.gov.

Recommended citation: Dyer EA, Kansagara D, McInnes DK, Freeman M, Woods S. Mobile Applications and Internet-based Approaches for Supporting Non-professional Caregivers: A Systematic Review. VA-ESP Project #05-225; 2012.

This report is based on research conducted by the Evidence-based Synthesis Program (ESP) Center located at the Portland VA Medical Center, Portland OR funded by the Department of Veterans Affairs, Veterans Health Administration, Office of Research and Development, Quality Enhancement Research Initiative. The findings and conclusions in this document are those of the author(s) who are responsible for its contents; the findings and conclusions do not necessarily represent the views of the Department of Veterans Affairs or the United States government. Therefore, no statement in this article should be construed as an official position of the Department of Veterans Affairs. No investigators have any affiliations or financial involvement (e.g., employment, consultancies, honoraria, stock ownership or options, expert testimony, grants or patents received or pending, or royalties) that conflict with material presented in the report.

TABLE OF CONTENTS

EXECUTIVE SUMMARY
    Background 1
    Methods 1
    Results 2
    Discussion 4
    Conclusion 5

DEFINITIONS AND ABBREVIATIONS 6

INTRODUCTION 8

METHODS
    Topic Development 10
    Search Strategy 10
    Study Selection 10
    Data Abstraction 12
    Study Quality 12
    Data Synthesis 12

RESULTS
    Literature Flow 13

    Key Question #1. How does the use of consumer health information technologies (CHIT) by non-professional caregivers of adult patients with chronic illnesses or disability, or by such patients who rely on a non-professional caregiver, affect outcomes for caregivers, patients, clinical process measures, and healthcare utilization? 14

    Key Question #2. What lessons can be learned from studies evaluating consumer health information technologies that specifically target the parents/caregivers of children? 28

    Key Question #3. What are the major gaps in the consumer health information technology literature serving non-professional caregivers of adult patients with regards to technology development, availability, and/or evaluation? 38

DISCUSSION 42
    Limitations 45
    Conclusion 45

REFERENCES 48

TABLES

Table 1. Characteristics and findings of studies of consumer health information technology interventions to support non-professional caregivers of adults with chronic illness or disability, stratified by care-recipient population 15

Table 2. Characteristics and findings of studies of consumer health information technology interventions to support non-professional caregivers of children with chronic illness or disability 31

Table 3. Summary of the functionalities available in health informatics interventions to support non-professional caregivers, stratified by care-recipient population 39

FIGURE

Figure 1. Literature Flow 13

APPENDIX A. SEARCH STRATEGY 55

APPENDIX B. INCLUSION/EXCLUSION CRITERIA 56

EXECUTIVE SUMMARY

BACKGROUND

Non-professional caregivers are an important source of physical, emotional and other support to ill or injured Veterans. With an increasing number of Veterans who require care and assistance for traumatic brain injuries (TBI), physical impairments, or other debilitating disorders such as post-traumatic stress (PTSD) and dementia, there is a greater growing demand for spouses, parents or other family members and friends to assume the role of caregiver. Electronic health applications and tools are increasingly available and have the potential to facilitate caregiving outside of traditional healthcare settings, especially in the context of the rising use of smartphones and mobile technologies. Lessons learned from prior consumer health information technology (CHIT) interventions could help inform the development of health-related mobile applications. CHIT applications are defined as electronic tools or technologies intended for use by consumers, by patients or family members, that interact directly with users for the management of their health or healthcare, and in which data, information, or other recommendations are tailored and/or individualized; the system may or may not link to a health professional or health system services. The Veterans Health Administration (VA) is currently developing mobile applications intended for use by seriously injured post-9/11 Veterans and their family caregivers enrolled in the Comprehensive Assistance for Family Caregivers program. This report was requested on behalf of the VA offices that are developing these mobile tools. The objectives of this report are the following: 1) to identify studies of CHIT applications that aim to support the needs of caregivers; 2) examine the usage and effects of CHIT applications on caregiver burden outcomes, and patient outcomes, clinical process measures, and healthcare utilization of interest; 3) discuss parallels that can be drawn from pediatric literature, and 4) identify gaps in the literature.

The key questions addressed by this systematic review are as follows:

Key Question #1. How does the use of consumer health information technologies (CHIT) by non-professional caregivers of adult patients with chronic illnesses or disability, or by such patients who rely on a non-professional caregiver, affect outcomes for caregivers, patients, clinical process measures, and healthcare utilization?

Key Question #2. What lessons can be learned from studies evaluating consumer health information technologies that specifically target the parents/caregivers of children?

Key Question #3. What are the major gaps in the consumer health information technology literature serving non-professional caregivers of adult patients with regards to technology development, availability, and/or evaluation?

METHODS

We conducted searches of multiple databases (MEDLINE® via PubMed®, Embase®, IEEE Xplore, AMIA Symposium Proceedings, Healthcare Information and Management Systems Conferences, Med 2.0, and Health 2.0) using terms for non-professional caregivers and mobile applications, including but not limited to terms for handheld/tablet computers, wireless/mobile technology, iPad, cellular/mobile/android/smart phone, m-health, Internet based, SMS, text messaging, and informatics application. We obtained additional articles from systematic reviews, reference lists of pertinent studies, reviews, editorials, and by consulting experts. Reviewers trained in the critical analysis of literature assessed the titles and abstracts for relevance, and retrieved full-text articles for further review. We included studies if they utilized patient-facing and/or caregiver-facing interactive computerized health information technology, regardless of whether the device used in the study was mobile (smartphone, tablet, etc.) or stationary (desktop). We excluded non-interactive healthcare technology such as health education materials that are passively used. Given the broad scope of this topic as well as the presence of other reviews, we excluded studies focused on telephony, interactive-voice-response, synchronous telehealth interventions, and fixed home-monitoring technologies such as smart-homes, vitals-monitoring, GPS and other location-monitoring, and monitoring for patient falls.

We compiled a narrative synthesis of findings, highlighting studies that evaluated the effects on caregiver outcomes, patient outcomes, processes, healthcare utilization and describe the common characteristics and themes that emerged across studies and disease categories.

RESULTS

We reviewed 2,605 titles and abstracts from the electronic search, and identified 16 additional references through manual searching of reference lists or from input from technical advisors.

After applying inclusion/exclusion criteria at the abstract level, 388 full-text articles were reviewed. Of the full-text articles, we rejected 331 that did not meet our inclusion criteria.

Key Question #1. How does the use of consumer health information technologies (CHIT) by non-professional caregivers of adult patients with chronic illnesses or disability, or by such patients who rely on a non-professional caregiver, affect outcomes for caregivers, patients, clinical process measures, and healthcare utilization?

We included 31 publications reporting on 22 CHIT interventions that were being developed, piloted, or evaluated for their effects on caregiver outcomes, patient outcomes, healthcare utilization, or process measures. Of these, there were five RCTs. The remaining studies consisted of feasibility studies, usability studies, pilot tests, qualitative studies, and quasi-experimental studies. The small sample size, variety of outcomes measured, diversity of interventions, and methodologic weaknesses of this body of evidence preclude any definitive assessment of health outcome or utilization effects of CHIT. There was little data to inform the effects of CHIT on clinical process measures.

The majority of articles described interventions that provided educational content and one of several communication modalities: either online peer support groups, online access to providers through email, or general disease information and education.

Studies consistently found that the online peer support groups and chat rooms were both the most-used and most-valued components of any given website, application, or intervention. The asynchronous nature of these online communications facilitates participation in support groups by mitigating some of the barriers of travel time, geographic separation, and competing priorities. In some studies, online communications provided access to a diversity of peers and clinicians that would otherwise not be available in many communities, particularly smaller town and rural environs. Anonymity was often perceived by users as an important feature of online support groups.

Several studies described how technical barriers or lack of familiarity with technology could limit accessibility of the intervention. Despite the numerous potential technical barriers, few studies reported the amount of technical assistance and training provided to users. Researchers speculated that older caregivers may be less likely to benefit from mobile applications because they are less likely to be users of handheld technology. A survey conducted in 2012 determined that while 70 percent of persons aged 65+ now own a cell phone, only 16 percent use their cell phone to access the Internet. Older caregivers may therefore require training in the use of the device or application, and may also benefit from applications with special accommodations for aging vision and manual dexterity, and their own chronic illness burden. Accommodations for language preference may enhance the utility of mobile applications for immigrant caregivers. Of note, no studies found that security or privacy concerns were a barrier to use of technology.

Key Question #2. What lessons can be learned from studies evaluating consumer health information technologies that specifically target the parents/caregivers of children?

We found 26 studies of 22 CHIT interventions in a variety of pediatric populations describing caregiver involvement with the intervention and/or caregiver outcomes. In all cases, parents were the caregivers being described. Cancer (4 interventions), traumatic brain injury (3 interventions), and diabetes (2 interventions) were the most common target conditions.

The largest group of studies described a multi-component intervention for children with traumatic brain injury and their parents, in which educational material was presented in interactive web sessions. The intervention was associated with reduced rates of parental anxiety and depression in three small, unblinded trials.

A larger trial involving asthma patients found that an intensive web-based intervention designed to improve parental and child knowledge of asthma reduced emergency room utilization. This intervention involved 44 animated lessons many covering real-life scenarios related to disease management and treatment adherence. Questions checked the user's comprehension.

Several studies also examined the role of online peer communication strategies. Parental users described benefits of peer support such as lowering the sense of isolation. While improving parental coping in some instances, users also pointed out the large volume of off-topic posts and posts about losing seriously ill children were detracting features.

Two studies evaluated text messaging interventions. One small trial in liver transplant patients found that a text-message medication reminder system involving children and parents reduced rates of biopsy-proven rejection. Another very large trial found that a simple text-message intervention in which parents received up to five weekly text messages increased influenza vaccination rates in a low-income population

Key Question #3. What are the major gaps in the consumer health information technology literature serving non-professional caregivers of adult patients with regards to technology development, availability, and/or evaluation?

The CHIT literature reflects a relatively new, developing field. Most studies described interventions in early development (ten studies) or pilot-tested (five studies) on a small scale. Only six studies were developed to evaluate health outcomes, but most of these were relatively small studies. There is a dearth of literature describing the health outcome effects of CHIT in larger populations. Some of the larger studies involved interventions, such as text messaging, which might be logistically simpler to deploy and test on a large scale. Almost no studies evaluated the actual implementation of interventions that had already been tested and found to be efficacious.

Reviewed studies were also not designed to develop a contextual understanding of the use of the intervention technology. At this time, there is not information to assess how these interventions fit into the day-to-day lives of caregivers. Additionally, there is relatively little information about how caregiver demographic characteristics impact the user experience. These are promising areas for future research; however, additional research is needed. For example, studies are needed to assess usage of mobile applications over time and to determine the most effective types of information, skills, and support that are needed to improve caregiver and patient outcomes.

The question of whether technology implementations should be designed for the caregiver or the patient as the end user is not answerable from the current literature, and may be best addressed by expert opinion and consensus.

DISCUSSION

There is a growing literature of CHIT interventions developed and tested for non-professional caregivers. Overall, a broad diversity of interventions has been identified, but the literature is insufficient to conclusively determine the effects of CHIT on caregiver/patient, healthcare utilization, or clinical process measure outcomes for a particular function or a specific condition. There is some evidence that CHIT interventions that target skill-building and stress reduction can be effective. Peer support and communication were the most commonly used intervention components; these functionalities were usually perceived as highly valuable. Though formal usability testing was not described in most studies, many studies described usage in more informal ways. Overall, the perceived utility of various technologies and their usage appeared to vary depending upon the caregiver target population. Some, but not all, studies described a user-centered design process. This may be particularly important for interventions targeting caregivers since they are burdened with self-care and the care of others, and the technology needs to fit into an often busy workflow.

It is unclear what CHIT interventions should be the focus of development in upcoming years. Multimodality interventions that combine different types of functions, applications, and devices (e.g., Internet, smart phones, text-messaging) may prove to be the most practical, given the rapid changes occurring in consumer technology development. Interventions focused on social support may reduce caregiver strain. Interventions, such as text messaging designed for cell phones without Internet, can reach large and low-income populations, and may be able to improve specific health behaviors. No studies described integration of CHIT tools with the healthcare provider's electronic medical record. A move toward greater interoperability could offer caregivers a valuable opportunity to access their care-recipients' personal health data, as well as to input information that could be used by clinicians such as home medications, side effects, and patient symptoms.

CONCLUSION

There is a growing literature of CHIT interventions developed and tested for non-professional caregivers. Overall, a broad diversity of interventions has been identified; the majority were multi-component online tools intended to improve knowledge, skills and coping, and provide social support of caregivers. Many of these multi-component interventions offered communication functions such as online peer support groups, email access to clinicians such as nurse specialists, "ask an expert" forum where questions are answered, informational tools such as online libraries and consumer guides to specific diseases, and educational content promoting stress-relief, wellbeing, and coping skills. Given the heterogeneity of interventions and measured outcomes, as well as of the evaluative methodologies used, it is difficult to draw over-arching conclusions regarding the impact of these technologies on caregiver, patient, or utilization outcomes. Nevertheless, lessons learned about usability and user experience from these studies may offer some valuable insight to help guide ongoing CHIT development.

DEFINITIONS AND ABBREVIATIONS

The following abbreviations are used throughout this document:

ACTION	Assisting Carers using Telematics Interventions to meet Older Persons' Needs
AD	Alzheimer's disease
ADHD	Attention deficit and hyperactivity disorder
BSFC	Burden Scale for Family Caregivers
BSI	Brief Symptom Inventory
CAI	Caregiver Appraisal Inventory
CG	Caregiver, non-professional family members, friends, or community members
CHESS	Comprehensive Health Enhancement Support System
CHIT	Consumer health information technologies, defined as interactive technologies that provide targeted or tailored health information and/or self-management tools or applications designed to support consumers' management of their health, health care, or health information
CR	Care-receiver/care-recipient, whether adult, child, or patient
CSES	Caregiver Self-Efficacy Scale
CSP	Customized Sleep Profile
CVA	Cerebrovascular accident, stroke
ER	Emergency room
HPN	Home Parenteral Nutrition
ICSS	Internet-based Caregiver Support Service
ICT	Information Computing Technology
ICU	Intensive care unit
IRC	Internet resources
IVR	Interactive voice response
KQ	Key question
NR	Not reported
OFPS	Online Family Problem-Solving
PCP	Primary care physician
PDA	Personal digital assistant
PDF	Portable Document Format, a file format used to represent documents for display on computers, smartphones and tablets
PIES	Prostate Interactive Education System

PTSD	Post-traumatic stress disorder
QOL	Quality of life
RCT	Randomized controlled trial
SCL-90	Symptom Checklist-90
SMS	Short Message Service, a protocol that supports text messaging for mobile phones
SNF	Skilled nursing facility
SRG	Stress-Related Growth
SUS	System Usability Scale
SWLS	Satisfaction with Life Scale
TBI	Traumatic brain injury
TOPS	Teen Online Problem Solving
Tx	Treatment
VA	Veterans Affairs, United States Department of
VHA	Veterans Health Administration
WAMMI	Website Analysis and Measurement Inventory
WECARE	Web Enabled Caregiver Access to Resources and Education

EVIDENCE REPORT

INTRODUCTION

The Department of Veterans Affairs (VA) recognizes the essential contribution of non-professional caregivers, who are an important source of physical, emotional and other support to ill or injured Veterans, including facilitating the ability for Veterans to remain in their homes. With the increased numbers of Veterans who require care and assistance for traumatic brain injuries (TBI), physical impairments, serious mental illness, and dementia there is a growing demand for spouses, parents or other family members and friends to assume the role of caregiver. Given the responsibility and diversity of tasks, and the ever-increasing reliance upon them by the healthcare system, caregivers themselves face impacts on their own quality of life, physical and mental wellbeing, and ability to manage their own healthcare needs. These impacts have been shown to be more frequent and severe for the caregivers of patients with illnesses such as dementia, neurologic disorders, and paralysis and likely have implications for Veterans' health status as well.

Health information technology advocates have long heralded the benefits of computerized tools used by patients and families for the delivery of healthcare information, education, and behavioral interventions. Opportunities for electronic health-related tools to engage patients in their healthcare and improve their health continue to increase as the consumer technology market expands rapidly and Internet penetration rises. However, the practical value and actual use of tools is challenged by a number of factors.[1-3] To be utilized as intended, consumer health information technology (CHIT) needs to be perceived as valuable, convenient, and relatively intuitive to use. Finally, these tools need to "fit" into an individual's workflow; for a patient with a medical condition, this represents seamless integration into one's activities of daily living.[4]

While a patient may not have access to technology, a loved one or caregiver could potentially access electronic information and tools on a patient's behalf. It is estimated that 34 to 52 million American adults provide home caregiving to another individual at some point in any given year.[5] Non-professional caregivers are typically not members of a licensed profession such as nursing, medicine, social work or psychology; instead, they are often family members or friends who either volunteer or work for small wages in order to coordinate care for the patient. Caregiver tasks range from basic (meal preparation, transportation to appointment) to more skilled (assistance with physical transfer, healthcare coordination, medication dispensing) and often require non-traditional work hours. Caregivers, in fact, increasingly look to the Internet for support and assistance with these tasks. According to Pew Internet & American Life national surveys, nearly half of those looking for health information online reported that their last search was on behalf of someone else.[6] In the same surveys, 70 percent to 80 percent of caregivers sought health information online, and 26 percent sought peer support online with other caregivers.[7]

Gaps remain in technology access across populations. Internet access continues to climb among young and middle-aged adults, yet those aged 65 and older with less than a high school education or living in a rural area continue to have lower rates of access.[8] Yet gaps in access continue to narrow and consumer demand for connecting to online information increases. Internet access increased from 46 percent of all U.S. adults in 2000, to 78 percent in 2010. Veterans and non-Veterans use the Internet at the same rate.[9] A total of 83 percent of adults now own a cell phone, with 77 percent ownership among those with an annual income under $30,000, and 56 percent among those aged 65 and older. Notably, the proportion of black or non-white Hispanic adults who own a cell phone was higher than the general population (44 versus 35 percent) as of May, 2011.[8]

The Veterans Health Administration (VHA) is developing applications for mobile devices intended for use by caregivers of chronically ill or disabled Veterans. The objective of this report is to identify studies of consumer health information technology applications that aim to support the needs of non-professional caregivers, examine the usage and effects of CHIT applications on caregiver burden and patient outcomes of interest, and identify gaps in the literature. Because some of the earliest research in caregiver needs and support is in pediatric populations, we also reviewed the pediatric literature to evaluate potential caregiver technology applications that may be further advanced or more rigorously evaluated than in the literature pertaining to caregivers of adult patients, and discuss parallels that can be drawn from pediatric literature.

METHODS

TOPIC DEVELOPMENT

The topic was nominated by the Office of Informatics and Analytics. The research questions for this systematic review were developed after a topic refinement process that included consultation between investigators, stakeholders, and content experts.

Key Question #1. How does the use of consumer health information technologies (CHIT) by non-professional caregivers of adult patients with chronic illnesses or disability, or by such patients who rely on a non-professional caregiver, affect the following outcomes:
    a. Caregiver-centered outcomes?
    b. Patient-centered outcomes?
    c. Process measures?
    d. Healthcare utilization outcomes?

Key Question #2. What lessons can be learned from studies evaluating consumer health information technologies (CHIT) that specifically target the parents/caregivers of children?

Key Question #3. What are the major gaps in the consumer health information technology literature serving non-professional caregivers of adult patients with regards to technology development, availability, and/or evaluation?

SEARCH STRATEGY

To systematically identify relevant articles, a research librarian conducted electronic searches of multiple databases (MEDLINE® via PubMed®, Embase®, IEEE Xplore, AMIA Symposium Proceedings, Healthcare Information and Management Systems Conferences, Med 2.0, and Health 2.0) using terms for non-professional caregivers and mobile applications, including but not limited to terms for handheld/tablet computers, Internet based, wireless/mobile technology, iPad, cellular/mobile/android/smart phone, m-health, SMS, text messaging, and informatics application. Appendix A shows the search strategy and the initial yields from each database. We obtained additional articles from systematic reviews, reference lists of pertinent studies, reviews, editorials, and by consulting experts.

We conducted a primary review of the literature yielded by the electronic search, and manually screened the bibliographies of included primary studies and any systematic or nonsystematic reviews that were identified.

STUDY SELECTION

Reviewers trained in the critical analysis of literature assessed the titles and abstracts for relevance. English-language articles included at the abstract stage underwent full-text screening by one investigator (ED, KM, MF, or DK), using prespecified inclusion criteria (Appendix B). We included studies either specifically enrolling a cohort of adult, non-professional, non-robot caregivers of adult patients (KQ1) or children (KQ2) with chronic illnesses or disabilities, or reporting caregiver outcomes. As this was an exploratory review and we anticipated few controlled trials would have been published, we did not limit by study design. We defined interventions and outcomes of interest as follows:

Interventions

Health information technologies are not currently limited by the device or operating system on which the function is available. We therefore considered technologies, applications, or functions that could be used via desktop computer, tablet computer, cell phone, smart phone, and/or personal digital assistant (PDA).

For the purposes of this report, studies were included if they utilized patient-facing and/or caregiver-facing interactive computerized health information technology. Such CHIT interventions include one or more of the applications listed in the taxonomy below:

- Education/skills: education and skill-building, such as topic-specific information, coaching modules, Question & Answer libraries, community resource information
- Self-care: decision aids, self-assessment with feedback, self-monitoring of conditions or care, patient portal access to electronic health record data
- Peer-to-peer communication: online forums, bulletin boards, listserv, email, chat and/or online support groups, with or without health professional moderation
- Caregiver-to-professional communication: secure messaging, email, chat or online forums with study staff or health professionals
- Patient-to-caregiver communication: tools that facilitate communication between caregivers, family members and care-recipients
- System transactions: transactional tools with the healthcare systems, such as medication refills, appointment requests
- Reminders: emails or text messages (SMS) to patient or caregiver on a specific issue, for example: medication reminders, notifications, or prompts on recommended care

We excluded non-interactive healthcare technology such as health education materials that are passively used and essentially reproduce paper in a digital form. We also excluded technologies consisting of access to general information such as directions, phone numbers, benefits review, and available services.

Studies that involved only telephony, interactive-voice-response, or synchronous telehealth interventions only were excluded in the report. We also excluded fixed home-monitoring technologies such as smart-homes, vitals-monitoring, GPS and other location-monitoring, and monitoring systems for patient falls.

Outcomes

The outcomes of interest were as follows:

1) Caregiver-centered outcomes: caregiver satisfaction, caregiver burnout, caregiver quality of life scores, caregiver depression/anxiety scores.
2) Patient-centered outcomes: patient satisfaction, patient activation, functional status, quality of life; quality of patient-caregiver relationship.

3) Process measures: clinician satisfaction; caregiver perceptions of mobile technologies; usage, usability, and barriers to usage of technologies/tools/applications; communication with healthcare providers.
4) Utilization outcomes: hospitalizations, ER visits, outpatient/PCP visits.

DATA ABSTRACTION

From the included studies, we abstracted data on the design and objectives of the study, and a brief description of the intervention. As there is not currently an agreed-upon convention for classifying the functional components of the CHIT interventions, we developed the seven categories described above. This taxonomy was adapted from multiple sources including: work performed by the Consumer Health Informatics Taxonomy Delphi study at Saint Louis University,[10] prior work by one of our co-investigators,[11] a systematic review performed by the Oregon Evidence-based Practice Center under contract to the Agency for Healthcare Research and Quality,[1] and a report developed by the VHA Health Informatics Initiative Patient-Facing Team.[12]

We characterized studies by research and implementation phase in categories adapted from the definitions put forth by the UK Medical Research Council on the development of complex interventions,[13] as follows:

- Development phase: studies that investigate intervention design-related outcomes (e.g., satisfaction, feasibility, usability) at an early stage of development.
- Pilot phase: studies that test user-related outcomes after the intervention has reached a relatively complete stage of development. Pilot studies are differentiated from evaluation studies if they have a small sample size (fewer than 50 participants) or if they do not report clinical outcomes.
- Testing and evaluation phase: studies that evaluate important user-related outcomes and have a sample size larger than 50 participants.

The categorization of studies by research and implementation phase is presented in Table 3.

STUDY QUALITY

Given the exploratory aims of the key questions, and because the yield of literature was largely descriptive, qualitative, and heterogeneous in a number of characteristics, we did not formally assess the internal validity of studies.

DATA SYNTHESIS

We compiled a narrative synthesis of findings, highlighting studies that evaluated caregiver outcomes and describing the common characteristics and themes that emerged across studies and disease categories.

RESULTS

LITERATURE FLOW

We reviewed 2,605 titles and abstracts from the electronic search, and identified an additional 16 studies from reviewing reference lists and consulting technical experts. After applying inclusion/exclusion criteria at the abstract level, 388 full-text articles were reviewed, as shown in Figure 1. Of the full-text articles, we rejected 331 that did not meet our inclusion criteria.

Figure 1. Literature Flow – Mobile Applications for Caregivers

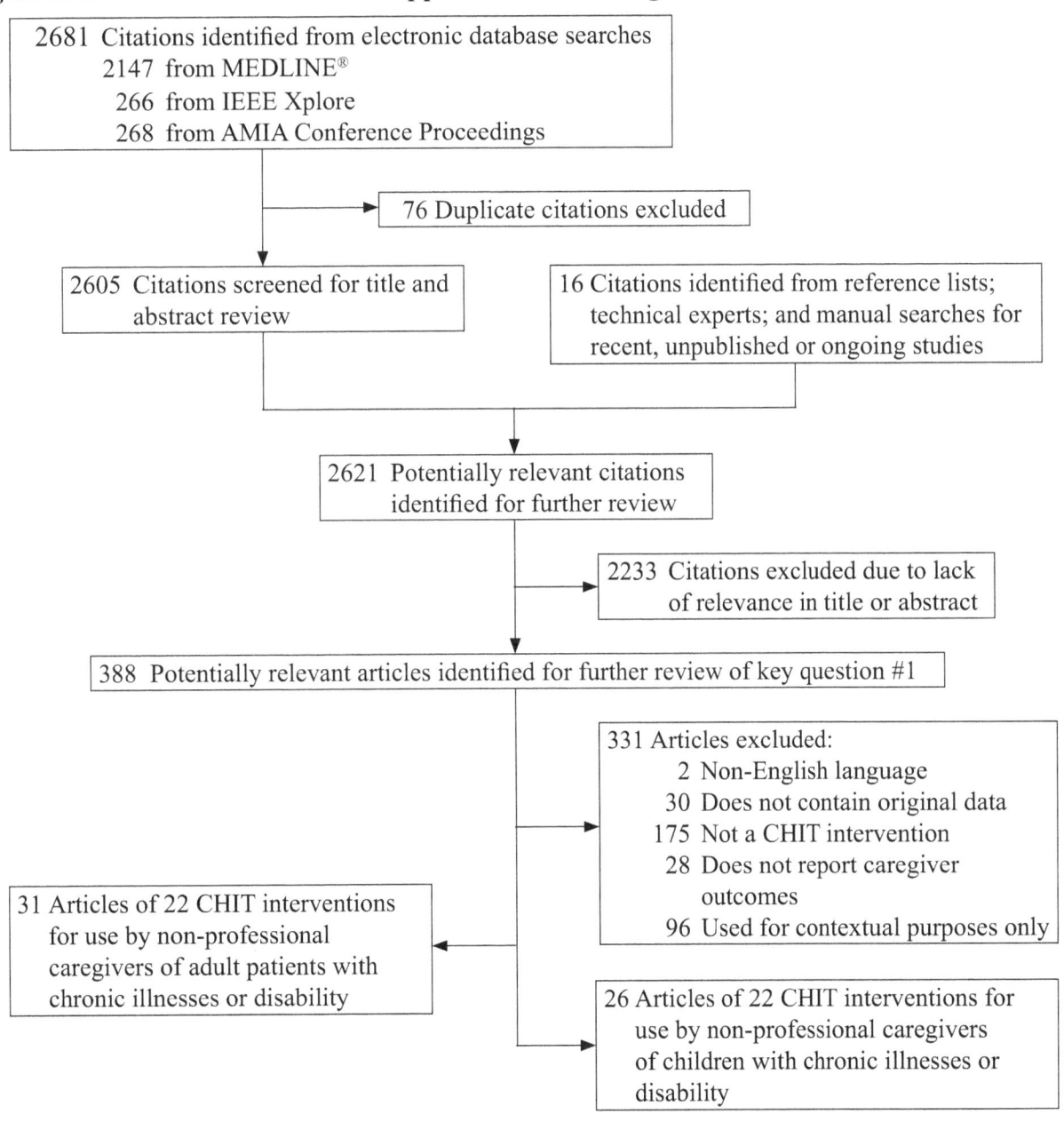

We included 31 publications reporting on 22 CHIT interventions that were being developed, piloted, or evaluated for their effects on caregiver outcomes, patient outcomes, healthcare utilization, or process measures.[14-43] Of these, there were five RCTs in seven publications;[16,19,20,23,26,27,35] the remaining studies consisted of feasibility studies, usability studies, pilot tests, qualitative studies, and quasi-experimental studies. We included 26 publications reporting on 22 interventions for caregivers of children with chronic illness or disability.[44-69] Twelve pediatric studies were RCTs.[46-49,55,57,59,63-65,67,70]

Studies on caregivers of adults and children with chronic illness or disability are shown in Tables 1 and 2, respectively. Table 3 shows the applications and functionality included in each intervention, and the phase of the interventions' lifecycle at the time of the study. Although many interventions contained non-interactive educational and resource materials, Table 3 also lists all interactive components of the intervention according to the classification taxonomy outlined previously.

KEY QUESTION #1. How does the use of consumer health information technologies (CHIT) by non-professional caregivers of adult patients with chronic illnesses or disability, or by such patients who rely on a non-professional caregiver, affect outcomes for caregivers, patients, clinical process measures, and healthcare utilization?

Summary of Findings

The majority of articles described interventions that provided education and one of several communication modalities: online peer support groups, online access to providers through email, or general disease information and education. Users expressed a desire for more social support and studies consistently found that the online peer support groups and chat-rooms were both the most-used and most-valued components of any given website, application, or intervention. The asynchronous nature of these online communications facilitates participation in support groups by mitigating some of the barriers of travel time, geographic separation, and competing priorities. Online communications provide access to peers and clinicians that would otherwise not be available in many communities, particularly smaller town and rural environs. Anonymity was often perceived by users as an important feature of online support groups.

Several studies described how technical barriers or lack of familiarity with technology could limit accessibility of the intervention. Despite the numerous potential technical barriers, few studies reported the amount of technical assistance and training provided to users. Older caregivers may be less likely to benefit from mobile applications because they are more likely to be non-users of handheld technology. Older caregivers may therefore require training in the use of the device or application, and may also benefit from applications with special accommodations for aging vision and manual dexterity, and their own chronic illness burden. Accommodations for language preference may enhance the utility of mobile applications for immigrant caregivers.

The characteristics and findings on interventions for caregivers of adult patients are shown in Table 1.

Table 1. Characteristics and findings of studies of consumer health information technology interventions to support non-professional caregivers of adults with chronic illness or disability, stratified by care-recipient population

Study design Sample size	Description of the intervention	Results	Comments on user experience (usability, access, training, satisfaction)
Alzheimer's disease or other cognitive impairment			
Quasi-experimental 23 families in Tx group, 19 families in control group Vehvilainen, 2002[14]	Alzheimer's Caregiver Internet Support System (ACISS) is a secure, interactive, Internet-based application targeted at supporting the medical, social, and psychological needs of AD caregivers and patients. ACISS networks caregivers, patients, a counselor from the Alzheimer's Association, and case managers from a geriatric care center.	• This pilot study collected data only on usage and user satisfaction over 6 months. • Tx participants (23 CGs) logged on to the site an average of 20x per month; Controls (19 CGs) logged on 10x per month. • User satisfaction was high: >75% said they would continue to use ACISS on a regular basis and suggest it to other CGs.	• Study author notes that users were enthusiastic about the system. • Participants with the added features of videoconferencing and multimedia behavior management tools logged on to the site twice as frequently as the standard features (reference information, secured messaging, chat, and message boards).
AlzOnline 21 family caregivers Glueckauf, 2004[71]	AlzOnline is an interactive Internet- and telephone-based education and support network that includes an Internet library, message board, chat room, and a series of 6 real-time interactive classes on positive caregiving. Caregivers who owned computer equipment that met the technical requirements for the interactive classes were eligible to participate. Classes were scheduled in small groups, typically 2-3 caregivers per group plus the class facilitator, once every 2-3 weeks for an average of 16 weeks.	21 of 40 enrolled caregivers completed the program. Comparison of pretest and posttest results: • Caregiving Self-Efficacy Scale: statistically significant ($p=0.02$) increases in all 3 subscales. • Stress-related Growth Scale: no significant change. • Caregiver Appraisal Inventory: significant reduction in subjective emotion burden subscale ($p=0.01$), no significant change in positive aspects or time burden subscales.	• Of 40 caregivers who matriculated in the Positive Caregiving class series, only 21 completed the program. • Primary reasons for dropout were work-related responsibilities, high involvement with caregiving obligations, and attending community-based support groups.
Development and pilot test Sample size not reported Becker, 2006[15]	PocketBuddy in-home virtual support system includes a PocketPC for reminders, monitoring of events and behaviors, and information support; and an integrated web page that updates automatically with information from the pocket computer.	• Technology in development. • Interviews with CG volunteers on desired features included quick timers and reminders for daily tasks, caregiving checklists, games for stress relief, virtual support group to communicate with other CGs. • Spousal caregivers who pilot-tested the device expressed satisfaction with the system and its potential usefulness.	• Technology is intended for older adult caregivers: Internet-based but uses a unique handheld device "PocketBuddy" with features designed to account for aging vision, cognition, motor skills, and hearing. • Pilot study included one 2-hour training session.
RCT 299 employed family caregivers Beauchamp, 2005[16]	Caregiver's Friend: Dealing with Dementia is a web-based multimedia intervention that provides tailored text material and videos that model positive caregiving strategies. Individual tailoring of materials and videos is achieved via a questionnaire that results in a list of links based on the patient's level of dementia and the caregiver's specific concerns. Program evaluation involved 299 employed family caregivers participating in a pretest/posttest RCT with a 3-day follow-up and a waitlist control condition.	• 150 Tx and 149 waitlist controls completed at pretest and 30-day follow-up. Surveys were used. • Tx CGs reported significant improvements in self-efficacy, intention to get support, and caregiver gain, stress, strain, depression, and anxiety, compared with controls. • Time spent in the program and composite gain score were significantly correlated ($r=30$, $p<0.001$). Average exposure to the program was 32 minutes.	Study author notes: with an average exposure of only 32 minutes to the program over the course of 1 month, 7 of 8 outcome measures yielded significantly positive results at 30-day follow-up.

Mobile Applications and Internet-based Approaches for Supporting Non-professional Caregivers

Study design Sample size	Description of the intervention	Results	Comments on user experience (usability, access, training, satisfaction)
Mixed-methods including usability study and interviews with 28 CGs Chiu, 2005[17] Chiu, 2009[18]	Internet-based support services (ICSS) for Chinese caregivers of people with Alzheimer disease (AD), has two components: 1) a CG information handbook, and 2) personalized email communication between client and a designated therapist (occupational therapy and/or social worker). The asynchronous email exchange occurred in a language of choice (English, Simplified Chinese, or Traditional Chinese).	• CGs were grouped by frequency of program use: non-users, occasional users (1-2 emails), and frequent users (3+ emails). • Primary outcome measure was BSFC (28-item Burden Scale for Family Caregivers). • Non-users (n=9) had increased BSFC scores at post-intervention (BSFC Change Score 5.22, 95%CI 10.24 to 0.20). • Occasional users (n=8) had minimal change in BSFC (0.50, 95%CI 10.86 to -9.86); frequent users (n=10) had a decrease in BSFC (-2.20, 95%CI -2.2 to 6.78). • Comparing non-users and frequent users, the difference in BSFC was significant (p=0.02).	• Chinese and English language options available. • CG language preferences between Chinese and English varied on the basis of communication mode: 60.7% preferring to write emails in English; while 60.7% were comfortable reading emails in either Chinese or English. • Almost all preferred being interviewed in Chinese.
RCT 51 CGs given access, 51 CG controls not given access Bass, 1998[19] Brennan, 1995[20]	ComputerLink is a computer network providing information, communication, and decision-support for caregivers of persons with Alzheimer's Disease. Communication included a nurse-facilitated bulletin board, and private email communication with the nurse for clinical expertise. The most widely used feature of ComputerLink was the communication component, which included a public bulletin board, private mail, and a nurse-facilitated Q&A segment. A separate feature was a 4-module electronic encyclopedia on Alzheimer's disease symptom management, services for patients and caregivers, and self-care for caregivers. 12-month RCT in which 51 caregivers were randomly assigned to have access to ComputerLink, and 51 to a control group that did not have access to ComputerLink. CGs received a 90-minute training session and coaching on the use of ComputerLink	• Tx (n=47) vs C (n=49) • Tx group had improved confidence in decision-making (p<0.01) between initial assessment and at 12 months. • ComputerLink did not significantly improve decision-making skills, or lead to decreased perceived social isolation among caregivers. • C-Link reduced strain in CGs who were initially more stressed and more frequently used the communication feature. Spouse CGs had reduced relationship strain vs controls. • Care-recipients in both group experienced similar declines in health status, although focus groups at the end of the study reflected perceived benefit of being able to communicate with peers and professionals at times of day that were convenient.	NR
Interviews on usability Sample size NR Kuwahara, 2004[21]	Network Interaction Therapy - Internet-based access to interactive communication between memory-impaired people, their family members, and volunteers. The multi-sensory system includes a large screen TV and a device for Internet communication, camera, microphone, and sensory media; an air cannon and a vibrator in the sofa to provide olfactory and haptic senses.	• Sample size not reported. In group interviews evaluating the need for and acceptance of the networked interaction therapy's capabilities, caregivers reacted positively to all of the intervention's capabilities except for networked interaction between memory-impaired people.	NR
Cancer			
User satisfaction survey 3,343 users Hill-Kayser, 2009[22]	OncoLife is a publicly accessible Internet-based tool for creation of individualized, detailed, comprehensive cancer survivorship care plans, providing surveillance recommendations for tumor recurrence, and guidelines for overall healthcare.	See usability comments.	>95% of non-provider users reported satisfaction levels of good to excellent. Average time to use tool by non-providers: 7.2 minutes. Of 3,343 users, only 12% of users were family or friends and not necessarily caregivers. Others were patients themselves or clinician providers.

Mobile Applications and Internet-based Approaches for Supporting Non-professional Caregivers

Study design Sample size	Description of the intervention	Results	Comments on user experience (usability, access, training, satisfaction)
RCT 285 lung cancer patient-caregiver dyads, 144 Tx, 141 controls Namkoong, 2011[23]	Comprehensive Health Enhancement Support System (CHESS) website: multicomponent interactive communication system included information services; peer and expert care communication services; and coaching/training services. Control group received usual care, a laptop computer with Internet access, and a list of high-quality, patient-directed lung cancer and palliative care. Tx group received access to the CHESS website with a laptop computer and Internet access.	Complicated statistics demonstrated that 2 years of CHESS access is associated with improvements in coping strategies compared to controls, and this is mediated through improved bonding. Measured bonding with 5 point Likert scale for feeling universality, obtaining emotional support, obtaining information, sharing feelings/fears, and building bonds. Positively correlated with appraisal-focused coping strategies and problem-focused coping strategies measured by "Brief Cope" which uses 5 point Likert scale to questions on "seeing it in a different light," "looking for something good," "concentrating on doing something about situation," "taking action to make it better," "getting help and advice".	Both Tx and control groups given laptop and Internet access and list of quality websites. Training NR. Researchers speculated that formal online discussion groups may have benefits not seen with informal web chat rooms due to closed membership, greater sense of belonging, common patient conditions (lung cancer), and linked educational and group communication components.
Descriptive analysis of themes in chat room postings Nolan, 2006[24]	Pancreatic cancer website - Internet-based cancer discussion and support group for pancreatic cancer patients and family members.	19% of postings addressed issues of spirituality, 6% of postings reported on death of a loved one which researchers suggest may be evidence of a utility in bereavement. One poster cited the chat room as a source of hope in contrast to her medical team. "Perhaps the anonymity of this venue is freeing."	Use: 600 total postings in 1 month. 68% of the postings explicitly stated relationship of poster to the patient. Of those, 83% (~325 postings) were posted by a family member, who was not necessarily a caregiver.
Focus group with 18 prostate cancer survivors and 15 spouses Diefenbach, 2004[25]	Prostate Interactive Education System (PIES) is a CD-ROM-based program that could be Internet based. It uses the metaphor of rooms in a virtual health center (i.e., reception area, a library, physician offices, group meeting room) to organize information. It allows for consultation with a surgeon and a radiologist; provides an extensive library of interactive videos of other patients' experiences undergoing the same treatment; and a system to assist patients with tailored decision-making. Dynamic system tailors information and summarizes what was learned when user exits.	See user experience comments. Caregiver subgroup analysis not performed.	• CD-ROM-based but can be Internet-ready according to authors. • Developed by a private vendor: Macromedia's Authorware. • 5 point Likert scale (5 high, 1 low). Very interested in site (4.7 +/- 0.6) and very useful (4.7 +/- 0.5). • 83% would prefer software over printed material. • Participants liked the virtual health center with rooms and offices concept, of accessing information in any order, and the mimicry of a human interaction.
Stroke			
RCT of 36 web users vs 37 non-web users Pierce, 2009[26] Steiner, 2008[27] Qualitative study of 13 CGs Keaton, 2004[28] Feasibility study of 9 CGs Pierce, 2004[29,30] Feasibility study Pierce, 2002[31]	Caring-Web was designed to provide easy and quick access to web-based education and support in home settings for caregivers of stroke survivors. The intervention has 4 components: 1) linked websites about stroke and caring; 2) customized educational information or tips specific to caregivers' needs; 3) an email forum to ask a nurse specialist and a rehab team private questions; 4) a non-structured nurse-facilitated email discussion among all participants.	• No difference in caregiver wellbeing after 1 year; measured by perceived depression (CES-D 20 item Likert scale, >15 is depression) at baseline: 12 v 11.3, and at 1 year: 12.3 v 9.0; also measured by life satisfaction (SWLS 5 item, measuring agreement with 5 statements) at baseline: 22.3 v 24.1 and at 1 year: 21.7 v 24.6. • Compared to participants in the control group, care-receivers in the intervention group had decreased healthcare use (self-reported provider visits, ER visits, readmission, SNF placements) decreased over time, with most of use in first 3 months, at which time users had less use. No difference in provider visits at one year 81 v 78, but at 3 months 156 v 188. Significant difference in ER visits 27 v 40 at one year (p=0.001) and readmissions 14 v 41 at 1 year (p=0.0005). • Caregiver emotional support was positively correlated with physical help, and with caregiver health (p<0.05). Results stable throughout study, not time-limited, thus caregiving is a continuous experience requiring continuous support.	• WebTV (Microsoft) or Internet-based. • Training provided and business hour telephone support. • 28 subjects did not have computers (and used webTV version), 23 had computers but needed Internet access. • Average use: 1-2hr/week. Total hits: 7,121; 102 messages to RN; 2,148 messages among subjects.

Mobile Applications and Internet-based Approaches for Supporting Non-professional Caregivers

Study design Sample size	Description of the intervention	Results	Comments on user experience (usability, access, training, satisfaction)
Mental Illness or traumatic brain injury			
Pilot and usability testing N=20 Stjernsward, 2011[32]	Exploratory study in which 20 participants tested a website for relatives of persons with depression for 10 weeks. The website comprises a diary (private and encrypted), and a supervised forum with members-only access.	See user experience comments for results. Usability optimized with an iterative design methodology.	4/20 dropped out. Usability formally assessed. System Usability Scale (SUS, 0-5 Likert scale, score 0-100, >70 is good): mean 78 (range 43-98).
Quasi-experimental feasibility study 26 families in Tx group vs 16 controls Glynn, 2010[33]	A web-based support and education intervention for key relatives of Veterans with schizophrenia or schizoaffective disorder, focusing on educational and support services to relatives, and also included a real-time professionally facilitated chat program in which closed cohorts of 5 to 6 relatives attended at specific times with a mental health professional over a 12-month period. "Proof of concept" feasibility trial compared 26 families of Veterans with schizophrenia or schizoaffective disorder, assigned to the online intervention with 16 controls receiving customary care.	• Brief Symptom Inventory (53 items, 0-4 Likert scale, no distress-extreme distress) did not change over time, and no difference between groups at 6 or 12 months. Family Attitude Scale (to assess patient-caregiver relationship stress, 30 items, 1-5 Likert scale): only measured in treatment group but did improve over time. Multidimensional Scale of Perceived Social Support (MSPSS, 12 items): only measured in treatment group and did not change. • Care-recipient hospitalizations: trend towards decreased admits in treatment group: 24% v 50%, X2 2.93, p<0.09.	Participants had to already have computer access at home. Participation: 79% completed year, attendance at weekly session: 59%. Attendance at optional sessions: 30%. 85% used the discussion boards. Usability formally assessed. 92% satisfied-extremely satisfied. Ease of use: 14% somewhat difficult-difficult. Unique challenges of online intervention: insuring access, addressing privacy concerns, managing emergencies adequately. Users had most difficulty with streaming videos and chats.
Feasibility study 19 CG-CR dyads Rotondi, 2005[34]	Web Enabled Caregiver Access to Resources and Education (WE CARE) has 7 modules: 1) an asynchronous online support group; 2) anonymously asking questions of experts; 3) a Q&A library; 4) a reference library of educational materials; 5) a calendar of community events; 6) a library of community resources; and 7) technical support. 19 dyads were provided access to the web intervention for 6 months, including computer and Internet service if needed. Caregivers were adult women who were the significant others of adult males with moderate to severe TBI.	• 75% very or extremely satisfied. • 94% very or extremely helpful. • 84% very or extremely supported. • Understanding evenly dispersed between moderately, very and extremely. • 38% not at all or a little motivated. • 14% moderately stressed still, 14% moderately lonely, 21% moderately angry, and 13% not at all to a little satisfying. • Used online support group most (69% of "hits" of > 1 minute duration). Average website visit of 15 minutes. Avg hits/user: 838 +/- 1015	The online support group was most used (69% of "hits" of > 1 minute duration) and valued module. Investigators noted challenges to use, including "lurking" without contributing, "flaming," and concerns as to whether electronic support groups provide equivalent emotional support.
RCT Tx group: 16 persons with schizophrenia and 11 CGs; Control group: 14 patients and 10 CGs Rotondi, 2005[35]	The Schizophrenia Guide web-based psycho-education program included 3 online therapy groups, ask-an-expert, library of previously asked questions, community activities and news items, educational materials. The RCT included 16 persons with schizophrenia and 11 family members or other informal support persons assigned to intervention; 14 patients and 10 caregivers assigned to usual care.	• Outcomes were measured at 3 and 6 months. • Reported lower perceived stress (p=0.04) among persons with schizophrenia in the intervention group compared to controls. • Reported trend toward higher perceived level of social support (p=0.06) among persons with schizophrenia in the intervention group compared to controls. • Caregiver/family member perceived stress and social support were not-significantly different between groups. • Total pages accessed: 17,292/3 months by persons with schizophrenia, 2,527/3 months by family members and informal support persons. • 1080 pages/schizophrenic user, 230 pages/caregiver, family member, or informal support person. • Most frequently used component: therapy groups. This was most highly valued part as well (44% said it was extremely valuable).	• Web-based. Adapted to "persons who had serious mental illnesses." • Usability formally assessed. Measured using 5 point ordinal scale (not at all – extremely) of helpfulness, understandability, value, ease of use. Among patients: 6% found it not at all easy, 70-80% found it moderately to extremely easy to use. 13% rarely or sometimes made sense, 88%, often or always made sense. Among caregivers: 0% not at all easy, 9% a little easy. 36% never or rarely made sense. Study author speculates that low engagement rates in psycho-education programs (14%) may be due to convenience and stigma.

Mobile Applications and Internet-based Approaches for Supporting Non-professional Caregivers

Study design Sample size	Description of the intervention	Results	Comments on user experience (usability, access, training, satisfaction)
Descriptive report with interview of 3 CGs; usability input from 2 case managers and 2 CGs Chiu, 2006[36]	Describes design of a digital device to facilitate caregiver planning of tasks and communication with other helpers and the care-recipient; speed up appointment decisions; simplify communication; improve access to resources; involve care-recipient; and adapt to changing support needs. Includes an electronic calendar, whiteboard, and dynamic user profiles.	See user experience comments.	Based on user needs, the device was designed to include speech recognition, large screen display, handwriting recognition, and touch screen.
Surgery and heart transplantation			
Pilot study 322 family members of patients undergoing surgery Huang, 2006[37]	To facilitate communication between the patient, hospital, and family, participants were sent between 2 and 5 SMS messages pre-, intra-, and post-operation. 322 family members of surgery patients received 685 text messages.	See user experience comments.	• Web-based, SMS to phone. • 92% strongly agreed that they were satisfied.
Pre-post intervention study 24 heart recipients and their family CGs vs 40 controls Dew, 2004[38]	An Internet-based psychosocial intervention program to improve mental health, quality of life, and medical compliance of heart transplant recipients and their families. Six components included post-transplant stress and medical regimen management workshops, monitored discussion groups, contact transplant team with non-emergency questions, Q&A library, healthy living tips, and resource/reference library. 24 heart recipients and their family caregivers were given access for 4 months, compared with a sequential control group of 40 heart recipients and their caregivers who did not have access to the intervention website.	Comparing pre- and post-test scores at 4 months: • Patient Mental Health over prior 2 weeks: as measured by the Symptom Checklist-90 (SCL-90), depression and anxiety scores decreased compared to controls (p=0.03, p=0.01). • Patient Anger-hostility score did not change over time and was not different between groups. • Caregiver Mental Health over prior 2 weeks (SCL-90): Anxiety score decreased compared to controls (p=0.05). Depression score decreased as well but was not different between groups. • Caregiver Anger-hostility score improved compared to controls (p=0.03). • Health-related QOL: as measured by the Short Form-36 (SF-36: measured physical functioning, pain, general health, energy/vitality, emotional wellbeing, role limitations due to physical health, role limitations due to emotional health, and social functioning), improved for both patients and caregivers. Was only administered to intervention group. • Self-reported medical compliance over prior 6 months (medication compliance, appointment attendance, consistency in lab work, physical exercise) • Greater use of website was associated with improved mental health and QOL. No change in compliance but a subgroup analysis of Medical regimen management workshop use was associated with increased compliance.	• Website accessibility: Able to login: 84%. Also 2 care-recipients and 1 caregiver were Internet novices and unable to overcome their hesitancy. • Frequency of use by caregivers: 41% monthly, 35% multiple per month, 23% weekly. • Avg duration: 15-30 minutes by 50%, >30 minutes by 12% • Ease of use: 93% very easy. • 50% never contributed to discussion group, 77% never asked an expert. • Discussion group most frequently used: 55% often, 20% sometimes. • Followed by Ask an expert 35% often, 45% sometimes, and Q&A library: 40% often, 35% sometimes.

Mobile Applications and Internet-based Approaches for Supporting Non-professional Caregivers

Study design Sample size	Description of the intervention	Results	Comments on user experience (usability, access, training, satisfaction)
Frail elderly, disabled NOS, and home parenteral nutrition			
Usability evaluation: 26 professional or informal CGs, and 242 first-time users of Ireland ACTION project Chambers, 2002[39] Cost-analysis study of 5 families in Swedish ACTION project Magnusson, 2005[40] Qualitative study of 34 families in Swedish ACTION project Magnusson, 2005[41]	Assisting Carers using Telematics Interventions to meet Older Persons' Needs (ACTION) is an interactive multimedia software application operated by a remote control instead of a keyboard/mouse; a television set instead of a computer monitor. The ICT-based support service enables family caregivers to access education, information, and support; to inform them about available choices and engage them in informed decision-making. ACTION has a range of multimedia caring programs accessed via PCs with access to education, expert care, Internet, and email access were included. Goal to help develop practical caring skills, information about available benefits and services, and develop ways of coping.	• Increased competence, satisfaction and sense of security in caregiving role per study, but data not provided. "Majority of 34 caregivers considered that their quality of life had increased." • Used a 40 question Likert scale (1 not at all - 5 a great deal) called PREP to measure caregivers preparedness, enrichment (rewards and satisfaction), and predictability. Mean score 3.1. Correlation noted between 7 caregivers who felt intervention was useful and had a PREP score >4. The 4 caregivers who felt it was not helpful had a PREP score <2. Data not presented, but state that intervention improved preparedness but not predictability of stressors implying that it did not reduce caregiver stress or burden. • Healthcare providers described feeling a shift in their role to empowering the caregiver. Time savings noted because care conferences held using videophone, rather than in-person.	• Large print, operated with remote control, using TV set (for increased familiarity). • Surveyed whether it was hard to read, images were clear, terminology difficult to understand (15%), screen layout confusing (11%), difficulty learning to use application, problems with navigating, instructions easy to follow, able to find information they desired, but 77% felt it took too many steps.[39] • 4 point Likert scale (4 high, 1 low). 88% gave application a 3 or 4 for ease of use, 68% 3 or 4 for satisfaction, 88% 3 or 4 for speed of use, 92% 3 or 4 for helpfulness. • Demonstration phase: average WAMMI for attractiveness 76, controllability 60, efficiency 71, helpfulness 74, learnability 67.5. • 5 out of 34 families did not use ACTION. • On scale from 1-10, caregivers reported usefulness of 6.4. Some users cited a lack of time as a barrier to use, due to pressures of caregiving. • TV based (for increased familiarity) with multimedia stored on a connected PC. Videophone software and camera provided that worked through television. Unclear if Internet was provided or if all users already had.
Qualitative evaluation of messages posted to national public online bulletin board over 3 months. 718 messages, 42 unique individuals Finn, 1999[42]	National public online bulletin board for patients with disabilities and their caregivers	• Computers assist people with disabilities that affect communication and slowed cognitive processes. Anonymity more important to this population, and finding peers. • Many messages had two or more purposes although evaluators only coded primary topic. Not focused on obtaining information alone: 55% socio-emotional support, 12% cathartic, 21% providing empathy, 11% chitchat, 14% problem solving. 1% taboo topics, 1% universality, <1% damaging statements.	Usage: 718 messages in 3 months, from 42 unique users.
Description of intervention, no primary data Fitzgerald, 2011[43]	The HPN Family Caregivers Website was developed to guide caregivers through the process of caring for themselves by establishing a caregiving routine, self-monitoring their mental and physical health, and practicing good sleep hygiene, while also managing the complexities of home care. Includes a self-assessment tool, diary checklist for recording daily routines and monitoring caregivers' emotions and energy, and tailored advice prompting mood-elevating activities when caregivers record feeling sad. Does not have online discussion group, but has "success stories" where users can submit their ideas/solutions, which are then edited by a curator and posted. Emphasizes importance of caregivers feeling connected to those providing health information.	See user experience comments.	Reports that users found it to be a "quality, reliable, and valid site".

Detailed findings

Our literature search identified 31 articles describing 22 CHIT interventions for caregivers supporting patients with a myriad of medical conditions. Interventions for caregivers of patients with Alzheimer's disease or dementia made up the largest group of studies (7 interventions published in 10 reports, of which 2 of these were RCTs examining intervention effects on caregiver outcomes).[14-21,71,72] The needs of caregivers for patients after cerebrovascular accident were targeted in six articles (1 intervention published in 1 RCT, 1 secondary-analysis, 1 observational study, and 3 feasibility studies);[26-31] caregivers of cancer patients in four articles (an RCT with lung cancer patient-caregiver dyads, and observational studies of pancreatic, prostate, and cancer in general);[22-25] caregivers of the frail elderly in four articles regarding one intervention,[39-41,73] with an additional one article addressing adults with "disabilities" that was not otherwise specified.[42] Two articles each addressed schizophrenia.[33,35] Two articles addressed traumatic brain injury.[34,36] The needs of caregivers for patients who were diagnosed with depression, receiving home-based parenteral nutrition, post cardiac transplant, or currently undergoing surgery were addressed in one article each.[32,37,38,43] Only one intervention was specifically evaluated in a VA population.[33] Details of the studies are found in Table 1.

The most commonly included applications and functionalities included education modules (12 studies); self-care aids (9 studies); peer-to-peer communication tools (13 studies); tools designed to improve caregiver-to-healthcare provider communication (11 studies). Only two studies examined email or text message reminder systems, two studies included tools to facilitate patient-caregiver communication, and no studies evaluated transactional tools such as online medication refills or appointment requests (Table 3).

In this section, we highlight studies that evaluated the effects on caregiver outcomes or evaluated specific populations relevant to the VA. We subsequently describe the common characteristics and themes that emerged across studies and disease categories.

Caregiver outcomes: Dementia population

One small RCT found that ComputerLink, a computer-based support network, reduced strain among caregivers.[20] ComputerLink provided a four-module electronic encyclopedia on Alzheimer's disease, but the more widely used feature was a communication component that included a public bulletin board, private mail, a nurse-facilitated Q&A segment, and private email communication with the nurse for clinical expertise. The study investigators installed computer equipment in the participants' homes and provided a 90-minute training session. After 12 months, ComputerLink was associated with reduced relationship strain among spousal caregivers compared with controls. Reduced strain was also observed among those caregivers who were initially more stressed and used ComputerLink communication features more frequently. Although the amount of care received did not differ between the treatment and control groups at the end of the study, caregivers perceived benefit from being able to communicate with peers and professionals at times of day that were convenient.[19]

AlzOnline, an Internet- and telephone-based education and support network, was associated with increases in perceived self-efficacy and reduced caregiver burden in a pre-/post-test study of 21 caregivers.[71] AlzOnline includes an Internet library, message board, expert forum, and a series of six live web- and telephone-based interactive classes on positive caregiving using cognitive-behavioral techniques. Caregivers who owned computer equipment that met the technical requirements for the interactive classes were eligible to participate. The average time to complete the series of classes was 16 weeks. Significant improvements were found on all three subscales of the Caregiver Self-Efficacy Scale (CSES), and the subjective emotional burden scale of the Caregiver Appraisal Inventory (CAI). No significant changes were found on the positive aspects or time burden subscales of the CAI, or on the Stress-Related Growth Scale (SRG). The study authors suggest that these differential findings may in part reflect the content of the intervention. The Positive Caregiving series of classes focused primarily on increasing skills in relaxation and the management of challenging caregiving situations, as well as enhancing perceptions of caregiver mastery and self-efficacy, with little emphasis on the rewards and emotional benefits of caregiving.[71]

Caregiver's Friend, a worksite-based support program, reduced caregiver strain in an RCT of 299 family caregivers who were also employed outside the home.[16] The Caregiver's Friend intervention was an Internet-based multimedia program that provided tailored text material and videos that modeled positive caregiving and coping strategies in a variety of scenarios. Individual tailoring of the online content was achievable via an interactive questionnaire that led to a menu of links based on the patient's level of dementia and the caregiver's specific concerns. Caregivers in the treatment group (n=150) were given access to Caregiver's Friend for 30 days. Pre-test and 30-day assessments were compared between caregivers in the treatment group and a waitlist control group (n=149). Compared with controls, caregivers in the treatment group reported significant improvements in self-efficacy; intention to get support; and caregiver gain, stress, strain, depression, and anxiety. Average exposure to the program was 32 minutes, and composite gain score was significantly correlated with time spent in the program (r=30, p<0.001).[16]

Caregiver outcomes: Lung cancer population

The Comprehensive Health Enhancement Support System (CHESS) program for patients with lung cancer and their caregivers improved caregiver coping strategies as measured in a two-year RCT of 285 patient-caregiver dyads.[23] The control group (N=141) received usual care, a laptop computer with Internet access, and a list of patient-oriented lung cancer and palliative care websites that the researchers felt to be of high-quality. The intervention group (N=144) was provided laptops and Internet connectivity, as well as access to the CHESS website that provides formal online discussion groups, communication with expert care, educational materials, FAQs, caregiver tips, health status tools, and decision aid tools, among others. Increased bonding among caregivers – suspected to be a result of the communication tools and online discussion groups – was found among CHESS users compared to controls (p<0.05). The increased bonding appeared to mediate improvements in both appraisal-focused coping ("cognitive efforts to define and redefine the personal meaning of the stressful situation," p<0.05) and problem-focused coping ("to modify or eliminate stressors by handling the reality of the demands," p<0.05) strategies as measured by a previously validated scoring tool called "Brief Cope." The mostly female (68%) caregiver users had a mean age of 55.6 years, and 50 percent had completed at least a college degree. The amount or frequency of use was not reported for the two-year study. Interestingly, only 42 percent of dyads completed the final survey. However, because the investigators were studying a population with advanced lung cancer, 84 percent of study dropouts were due to the death of the patient; thus, the high attrition rate does not appear to be indicative of use or usability obstacles.

Caregiver outcomes: Post-surgical population

A two-group prospective, pre-/post-test intervention study of post-heart transplant patients and their caregivers demonstrated improved caregiver outcomes in those who used an Internet-based website for four months.[38] The intervention group comprised 24 heart transplant recipients and their family caregivers with access to a website of educational resources and psychosocial interventions such as: online, self-paced workshops on post-transplant stress management and medication management (both of which included self-assessment tools, decision support, and tailored advice), clinician-moderated online discussion groups, email contact with transplant team members, a Q&A library, healthy living tips, and a resource library. The control group consisted of 40 heart transplant recipients and their caregivers who were enrolled in other non-Internet-based interventions at the same institution over a four-month period either immediately before or immediately after the present study. Mental health (depression, anxiety, and anger-hostility) was measured using the Symptom Checklist-90 (SCL-90), which assesses mental health over the past two weeks. Caregivers in the intervention group had significant improvements in both their anxiety and anger-hostility scores from pre-intervention to post-intervention compared to controls ($p=0.05$ and $p=0.03$, respectively). Caregiver depression scores also improved over time but were not significantly different between intervention and control groups. Health-related quality of life, as measured by the Short Form-36 (SF-36), improved for both patients and caregivers in the intervention group over time, but was not evaluated in controls. Finally, a subgroup analysis found that those patient/caregiver dyads in the intervention group who used a particular component of the website, an online workshop about medication management, had increased compliance as measured by frequency of completing recommended appointments and lab work. Similarly to other studies, the majority of caregivers were female (85%), married (85%), and Caucasian (90%); 50 percent had at least a high school education.

Caregiver outcomes: Veterans

Only one intervention was specifically evaluated in a VA population.[33] This was a prospective trial of a web-based intervention for relatives of Veterans with schizophrenia or schizoaffective disorder. It provided educational and support services to relatives, and included an online professionally-facilitated multi-family support group. The 26 family members in the intervention were compared to an historical control group of 16 family members who had received other support services in the four years prior to this study. They found that there was no difference between intervention and control groups in family members' measurement of distress using the Brief Symptom Inventory scoring tool. A measurement of stress between the family member and patient did improve over time in the intervention group, but was not measured in the control group. A trend towards decreased hospitalizations among care-recipients was noted in the intervention group compared to controls but was not significant (24% v 50%, X^2 2.93, $p<0.09$). Family members were predominantly female, with a mean age of 57 years old and an average of 14 years of education. Of note, they were not specifically caregivers for the VA patient. Seventy-nine percent of family members completed the year-long program, 85 percent also used the online discussion boards, and there was an average attendance of 59 percent at the weekly online family support group sessions.

Effects on healthcare utilization: Stroke population

The Caring~Web studies were notable for evaluating healthcare utilization by care-recipients. In a three-month descriptive study of five caregivers of patients who had recently been discharged to home from a rehabilitation treatment center after a stroke, investigators measured the number of phone-calls to a clinician's office (range 1-4), appointments (range 2-3), emergency department visits (1), and hospital admissions (1).[31] In a subsequent evaluation, a one-year RCT demonstrated that self-reported, utilization of healthcare services was less compared to controls.[26] The intervention group consisted of caregivers of patients with a recent stroke (n=36) who were provided access to the Caring~Web application, a website with links to educational information on strokes and caregiving, tips for caregivers, an email link to solicit expert care from the institution's nurse specialist and a multi-disciplinary stroke rehabilitation team (consisting of a physician, pharmacist, dietician, social worker, and therapists), and an email discussion group facilitated by the nurse specialist. The control group comprised caregivers (n=37) that would not be using the web. All recruited caregivers were Internet novices. After one year, the intervention group's care-recipients had 33 percent less emergency department visits (p=0.001), and 66 percent less hospital admissions (p=0.0005) compared to the patients of caregivers in the control group. Fewer clinician provider outpatient visits were noted at three months (156 vs 188 visits), but this had become non-significant at one year of follow-up. These findings suggest that care-recipients in the intervention group received more appropriate or timely care, thus preventing emergency department visits and subsequent hospital admissions, perhaps due to their caregivers having improved access to information or closer communication with clinician providers as a result of the Caring~Web intervention. Again, caregivers were primarily female (75%), the spouses of the care-receiver (70%), with a mean age of 55 years, and ~90 percent had achieved a high school education or greater.

Common CHIT intervention characteristics among studies

Regarding the types of caregiver needs that were addressed, the majority of articles described interventions that provided one of several communication modalities: either online peer support groups, online access to providers through email or SMS/texting, or general disease information and education. The majority of interventions provided all three of these communication modalities in a single site/application, making it difficult to identify exactly which component of the intervention accounted for the outcomes.[14,19,20,23,25,27,32-36,38,74]

Online peer support groups and chat rooms, whether professionally moderated or not, were consistently found to be both the most-used and most-valued components of any given website, application, or intervention.[23,24,34,73,74] Even preliminary feasibility studies found that users expressed a desire for more social support and inter-personal communication, that presumably would be addressed with such an intervention.[31] Analysis of conversational themes from one online chat room found that users frequently acknowledged a perceived benefit both from participating in a community of peers, and knowing that other caregivers faced similar challenges.[30] Multiple studies speculated that, compared to in-person support groups, online peer support groups improved access and anonymity. Clearly, online, asynchronous communication allows users to participate in a support group while mitigating some of the barriers of travel time, geographic separation, and time constraints from competing priorities. Evaluations of Caring~Web also pointed out that online communications provide access to a diversity of peers and clinicians that would otherwise not be available in many communities, particularly smaller town and rural environs.[28,30] Anonymity was often considered an important feature to users of online support groups, and several authors speculated that caregivers and patients with chronic medical illnesses may have feelings of stigma or actual communication disabilities (hearing difficulties, slowed cognitive processes, etc.) that are overcome in faceless, asynchronous communication.[24,28,34,35,42]

CHIT interventions commonly allowed users to pose questions to a clinician, variously called "Ask an Expert/Nurse," "Expert Care," "Q&A," or "Frequently Asked Questions." Such communication with clinicians allowed users the opportunity to ask questions and, in many cases, the intervention included an online "library" of previously asked questions with the related responses. All of the interventions in adult caregivers and patients provided this functionality via email from the website; none used alternative technology such as SMS/text messagings. In the majority of interventions, the email was sent to a nurse specialist; although email access to other clinician experts was also described, including an Alzheimer's disease counselor and case manager,[14] occupational therapist and social worker.[17,18] Two interventions described in detail how a multidisciplinary team provided the expert care: the email went to a nurse coordinator who then consulted with the cardiac transplant team in one case,[38] or a team consisting of a physician, pharmacist, dietician, social worker, and therapists.[26,31] In the pediatrics literature, use of SMS/text messaging in the evaluated intervention was quite common perhaps due to researchers' perception that parents of young children were likely to be familiar with current mobile phone and computing technologies.

User-centered design

According to the Usability Professionals Association, User-centered Design is the approach to design that grounds the process in information about the people who will use the product.[75] The process focuses on the usability of the product or service, making sure that users can readily and effectively accomplish their tasks as intended. Usability is considered part of a wider concept of *user experience*, or the way an individual (user) feels about using a product or service. User experience highlights the experiential and affective value or other meaningful aspects of human interaction; and also includes perceptions of utility, ease of use and efficiency of the system. User experience can be dynamic and change over time as the circumstances change.

Usability

A limited number of studies assessed usability using formal tools and iterative design methods.[32,39] Chambers et al. used the Website Analysis and Measurement Inventory (WAMMI) to assess the initial implementation of the Assisting Carers using Telematics Interventions to meet Older Persons' Needs (ACTION) intervention.[39] They found that usability problems related to difficulty understanding terminology used on the website (15%), confusing screen layout (11%), challenges learning to use the application, and problems with navigation. More telling, 77 percent felt it took too many steps to reach information they desired. In an exploratory study of a Swedish website application to support the informal caregivers of patients with depression, Stjernsward et al. found that the 20 pilot users gave the application a mean System Usability Score of 78 (range 43-98), suggesting good usability overall (>70). However, notably 20 percent of users dropped-out of this exploratory study, which may indicate that some users were unable to continue using the application due to usability issues.

One pediatric study evaluated the usability of cystic fibrosis, diabetes, or arthritis portals by novice users.[54] Their approach illustrates some of the very simple and practical information such testing can yield. For instance, parents pointed out use of jargon and abbreviations as barriers to understanding information, and they wanted confirmation that communication with healthcare professionals was received.

The Caregiver Support Service, developed for Chinese Canadians and associated with decreased caregiver burden among frequent users, examined language preferences among 28 caregivers of patients with dementia.[17,18] Users could access a bilingual portal for caregiver information or email an occupational therapist and social worker. Most caregivers resided with the patient; the typical caregiver was female, aged 40 to 60, worked full-time, had a college education, was born outside of Canada and immigrated to Canada 10 to 20 years prior. Most care-recipients were the parents who co-resided with the CG. All spousal CGs invited to participate declined use of the email support service, and the study authors speculated that this may be a cohort effect associated with age.

A handheld device called PocketBuddy was developed for use by aging adult caregivers, with accommodations for poor vision, cognitive function, motor skills and hearing.[15] Features of the device include landscape mode for greater screen space, optional large font to improve readability, button lists, finger tapping, enlarged keyboard, audible cues, and multimodal support options. Various functions include assisting in caregiving activities, monitoring the well-being of both caregiver and care-recipient, and networking the caregiver with family and friends to actively involve others in the daily life of the caregiver and care-recipient. The device was pilot-tested by eight older adults (aged 65-89 years), including two spousal Alzheimer's disease caregivers. The caregivers expressed satisfaction with the system and its potential usefulness, though further details were not reported.[72]

ACTION caregiver users had a mean age of 70 years (range 47-88 years) and the technology was specifically designed to meet the needs of older adults, including large print to accommodate vision deficits.[39,41] The Prostate Interactive Education System (PIES) intervention to assist diagnosis and treatment decision-making found that 89 percent of users had no vision difficulties impacting ability to use technology, and 83 percent had no difficulty with using a mouse.[25]

In general, these studies highlight some notable barriers and accommodations necessary when considering use of technology interventions for older caregivers, whether deployed on mobile computer platforms or not. A demographic survey of cell phone Internet usage conducted by the Pew Research Center determined that seniors (aged 65+) had the lowest usage rate among any major demographic group. Although 70 percent of persons aged 65+ currently own a cell phone, only 16 percent of them use their phones to go online.[76] Older caregivers may require training in the use of the device or application, and may also benefit from applications with special accommodations for aging vision and manual dexterity. However, one study did note that streaming video applications that might accommodate older caregivers with vision or attention deficits was the component with which users were most likely to experience technical difficulties.[33] Accommodations for language preference may enhance the utility of mobile applications for immigrant caregivers.

User experience

A number of studies described the usage of the CHIT interventions through the lens of the caregiver or patient users. Many of these evaluations or qualitative descriptions were not primary goals of the study, yet offer important information related to their drivers or barriers to use. A few examples are illustrated here, across the adult and the pediatric literature.

The modality of tool or type of functionality offered was perceived to be important in a few studies. Among teens with traumatic brain injury and family members, the availability of audio recording enhanced the users' ability to relax and comprehend the written content.[67] Parents given the choice of a DVD or an Internet-based intervention after a child's injury felt that the web tool offered greater accessibility.[69]

Many studies offered peer-to-peer communication, which as described previously, achieved high satisfaction and use. Individual comments about peer communication tools provide glimpses into reasons for this user experience. Children with diabetes[58] and juvenile arthritis,[45] and their parents using a portal to communicate with peers received social support by "not feeling alone" and perceiving greater universality in their journey. Parents of children with cancer were positive about the convenience of communicating at any time, the ability to "vent" their feelings through words, and feeling less isolated knowing others were experiencing the same condition and issues.[50,51] Caregivers of patients with Alzheimer dementia reported that use of peer-peer communication was reassuring and led to greater self-efficacy as a caregiver.[18,20] While views of peer online peer support were overwhelmingly positive, some users described negative experiences. Parents of children with cancer felt stressed when another child died;[51] others were less satisfied if discussions "went off topic,"[51] or there were insufficient numbers of participants to achieve "critical mass".[32,50] Of note, although some groups were moderated by staff and others were not moderated, there were no comments about the effect of health professional moderation.

Some studies reviewed for this report also described the process and/or results of soliciting user participation in the development and design process. Parents and teens with juvenile arthritis provided valuable input during development, leading to improvements in website navigation and display of information, such as reducing ambiguity of medication information presented.[45] Parents of children with diabetes also pointed out problems with medical jargon and lack of information about normal values of laboratory data.[54] Caregivers of patients with depression found it important for developers to ensure there was clear descriptions of functions so as users would understand their value. These caregivers also pointed out that using real names on peer communication violated privacy; when reminded by the study team that real names were optional and described in the user instructions, users remarked that instructions usually were not read.[32]

Technical challenges

Technical barriers or lack of familiarity with technology were described in several studies as potentially limiting accessibility of the intervention. Dew found that 16 percent of would-be users were unable to login and thus never able to access the intervention.[38] Five of 34 families never used the ACTION intervention site due to technical difficulties.[40] Multiple studies documented that intended users of the implementation frequently did not have a computer, let alone Internet access; those who did were only minimally experienced in their use, and sometimes the caregivers' or care-recipients' hesitancy to use an unfamiliar technology could not be overcome;[25,26,32,34,38] however, these articles are through 2009 and thus might not represent current users' computer and Internet experiences. Both the Caring~Web[26,27] and ACTION [39,40] interventions were designed for use with a standard television and remote control (using Microsoft's WebTV product) in order to increase user familiarity and overcome barriers, such as computer and Internet literacy. Of note, no studies found that security or privacy concerns were a barrier to use of technology.

One conference abstract described a qualitative study analyzing reasons why an electronic care management tool for type 1 diabetics failed to meet functionality expectations. Investigators conducted key informant interviews and surveys of patients and their parents which revealed several points of failure, including lack of patient or parent time/interest, glucometer malfunction, and lack of Internet service (especially for participants in rural settings).[57]

Few studies reported the amount of technical assistance and training provided to users. As part of the Caring~Web intervention, a technician installed the television software required or, in some cases, a computer and Internet connectivity, instructed caregivers and patients on its use, provided a paper-based support manual, and was available for technical assistance via phone throughout the study.[26,27] Families enrolled in the Online Family Problem-Solving (OFPS) intervention for children with TBI were given a computer, printer, and webcam, and extensive in-person training on use of the equipment.[66] In contrast, Chambers noted that during ACTION's Ireland implementation, staff had insufficient time to explain the system to users.[39] Not one study quantified the costs or amount of time that user training and ongoing support required; although, anecdotal experience suggests that these often surpass the initial capital investment of technology implementations.

KEY QUESTION #2. What lessons can be learned from studies evaluating consumer health information technologies (CHIT) that specifically target the parents/caregivers of children?

We found 26 studies of 22 CHIT interventions in a variety of pediatric populations describing caregiver involvement with the intervention and/or caregiver outcomes (Table 2). In all cases, parents were the caregivers being described. Cancer (4 interventions), traumatic brain injury (3 interventions), and diabetes (2 interventions) were the most common target conditions. The following sections describe examples of different intervention subtypes tested in pediatric populations.

Self-management education and enhancing caregiver-patient communication

A number of studies described interactive educational web-based interventions designed to help patients and their parents develop self-management skills for chronic illnesses such as TBI and asthma. The largest group of studies described a multi-component intervention for children with traumatic brain injury and their parents. The online family problem-solving (OFPS) intervention includes logistic and educational material presented in 12 distinct interactive web sessions. The family collectively completed each module, entering responses to questions posed by the program and receiving tailored feedback from the website. Completed exercises were stored online and reviewed by a therapist, who also conducted a synchronous online videoconferencing session with the family after each module was completed. A small, unblinded RCT found the OFPS was more effective than static Internet resources alone in reducing parental depression and anxiety, though it was impossible to separate the effects of the web intervention from the videoconferencing sessions. Of note, nearly half the parents had no more than a high school education suggesting the potential feasibility of a complex web-based intervention in populations with varied educational backgrounds.[64] The same group of investigators more recently developed a version of OFPS designed for adolescents and similarly found reduced parental depression and improved parent-child communication.[67,68] An earlier feasibility study of the OFPS intervention found that technical issues such as the type of webcam used and virus infection could affect intervention usability.[66]

One RCT of 228 children and their parents evaluated the effects of a multi-media Internet asthma education program compared to standard print/verbal education on child/parent disease knowledge, asthma symptoms and emergency room utilization.[46,47] The intervention, which included 44 vignettes designed to be reviewed in about one minute – suited to a child's attention span – increased child and parent knowledge of asthma, and was associated with significantly decreased ER utilization and asthma symptoms compared to control participants.

Peer communication

Caring for a chronically ill child can be anxiety-provoking and also isolating, as parents of healthy children may not understand their experience. Several studies examined the role of electronic peer communication strategies. Han et al. surveyed 73 parents about their experience with online support groups for parents of children with cancer.[51] Over three-quarters (77%) of parents highly valued the informational aspects of the support groups including information about the cancer itself and its treatment. While they also valued sharing experiences, receiving general support, venting feelings and gaining accessibility, they identified large volumes of often off-topic mail/posts and lack of face-to-face contact as drawbacks.

Demaso et al. evaluated a web-based tool for sharing personal stories about caring for children with cancer.[56] They found that on a seven-point scale, parents reported the application increased their understanding of their experience as a caregiver of a child with depression (mean rating of 5.4). In addition, 83 percent reported that the tool helped them to understand symptoms of pediatric depression. Families in this study also reported that they learned ways to cope with stressful circumstances.

System transactions, accessibility and efficiency

Some of the online tools reported gave 24-hour access to laboratory results, medication lists,[52,62] and secure messaging with providers.[53] This kind of access – for example, secure-messaging – was also seen as more efficient and less frustrating than playing telephone tag with clinicians.[53]

Two studies evaluated text messaging interventions. One examined the effects of an automated text message reminder system on medication adherence and transplant rejection rates in pediatric liver transplant patients.[60] Participants entered contact information online for patient and caregiver, medication information, and the desired time for alerts. Text messages were initially sent to the person responsible for medication administration (parents for younger children, and the patients themselves in older age groups); the caregiver was notified if a message confirming medication intake was not received within 30 minutes. A pre-/post-study of 41 children found significant improvement in immunosuppressive drug levels, and a reduction in biopsy-proven transplant rejection over one year. Though the impact of this simple intervention on health outcomes is promising, several issues including a high attrition rate (37%) which may raise concerns about the acceptability of this type of reminder system should be noted.

One large RCT examined an intervention to increase influenza vaccination rates in an urban, low-income pediatric and adolescent population in which parents received up to five weekly text messages.[59] The messages included educational information about the influenza vaccine – to reduce misconceptions – and information about Saturday flu vaccine clinics. Texts were personalized to include the child's name in the body of the text message. Both the intervention group and the control group received usual care, which was an automated telephone reminder. A higher proportion of intervention group (42.6%) received immunizations, compared to controls (39.9%) (relative rate ratio=1.09; CI=1.04-1.15, p=.001). This study demonstrated the feasibility of reaching significant numbers of parents/caregivers using text messaging. Though the absolute increase in vaccination rates was only three percent, given the low cost of texting, this is still likely to be a cost-effective intervention. Of note, the texts used multiple strategies aimed at reducing barriers to child vaccination: one was to inform about the vaccine, intended to reduce parent concerns about possible dangers from vaccination; a second was providing practical logistic information about the time and place for the vaccine clinics; and a third was a reminder function.

User experience

This information is summarized in Table 2 and in the "User experience" section under Key Question #1.

Mobile Applications and Internet-based Approaches for Supporting Non-professional Caregivers

Table 2. Characteristics and findings of studies of consumer health information technology interventions to support non-professional caregivers of children with chronic illness or disability

Pediatric population Study design Sample size	Description of the Intervention	Results	Findings on usability of technology
ADHD, newly diagnosed Survey on usability by parents or caretakers Convenience sample 195 completed pre-test 12 completed post-test Ossebaard, 2010[44]	Online treatment decision aid to help parents make decisions about the kind of care and treatment would be best for their child with ADHD.	• Poor response rate (only 12 completed both the pre- and post-test questionnaire, which were separated by 3 months). • In 3-month study period about 7,500 visited the online ADHD decision aid. • Small non-significant increase in decisional conflict (from mean=55 (SD=30) to 57 (27), p=0.94, and self-report knowledge (from 6.5 (1.9) to 6.7 (1.5), P=0.89. • Small non-significant decrease of the stage of decision-making (from 2.6 (1.1) to 2.2 (0.7), P=0.16. • The DA contributed to better preparation for decisions and facilitated decision-making. Satisfaction with the information received through the DA was moderate, and 60% felt that the information was too limited.	94% of respondents did not complete both questionnaires; the authors took this to indicate that the navigational flow and usability of the online decision aid might have been too complicated.
Arthritis, juvenile rheumatoid Interviews on usability 11 English-speaking teen-parent dyads, and 8 French-speaking dyads Stinson, 2010[45]	Interactive, web-based program composed of 12 modules including disease-specific education, self-management strategies, peer networking, and 2 modules designed to help parents promote healthy behavior in their teen children.	None; development phase.	• Few navigation errors. • Numerous presentation errors (mostly in finding medication links) - improved with corrections. • Control usage errors were also discovered and corrected. • Participants identified four types of design aesthetics as important: layout, navigation, visual assets, and visual appeal. 89% of teens and 95% of parents felt content was relevant. 74% teens and 79% parents felt content was trustworthy. • Participants suggested addition of videos/photos to demonstrate exercises would be helpful. • Adaptive and interactive features were highly rated (glossary, audio clips, PDFs, "Ask an Expert" discussion board). • Nearly all teens felt the discussion forums would be helpful, while only half the parents felt similarly.
Asthma RCT CGs of 228 children (n=121 in control; 107 intervention) Krishna, 2000[46] Krishna, 2003[47]	Interactive, multi-media, Internet education program with 44 vignettes that take less than 1 minute for child to complete. For children <7 years old, the parent used the program; for children 7-17, the child used the program while parents observed. Ten of the vignettes require the user to make a decision about a kind of behavior that is likely to affect asthma. Control received just the traditional educational information.	• Increased asthma knowledge between visit 1 and visit 3 was greater for the intervention groups than for controls for caregivers of children <7, Chi-sq=6.92, P<0.01; for caregivers of children 7-17 Chi-sq=7.21, P<0.01; for children 7-17 Chi-sq=11.71, P<0.01. • Respective increases for these intervention groups were from 47.9 (5.2) to 55.7 (4.3); 50.0 (5.6) to 55.4 (4.2); and 43.1 (6.8) to 53.1 (5.6). • Intervention group showed greater decrease in asthma symptom days. Decrease of 81 days for intervention vs. decrease of 51 for control, Chi-sq=6.7, P<0.01. • Intervention showed greater decrease in number of ER visits, 1.93 vs. 0.62, Chi-sq=5.1, P<0.01. • Intervention group also had lower average daily doses of inhaled corticosteroids, 434 μg vs. 754 μg, Chi-sq=7.3, P<0.01.	• Modified for children. Short vignettes of under a minute each (for shorter attention span). Users reported it was easy to use and navigate, interesting, and enjoyable. • Caregivers of children <7 and caregivers of children 7-17 reported easy to use (82% and 89% respectively), interesting (68% and 44%), enjoyable (41% and 33%), easy to navigate (82% and 67%), and will use again (86% and 67%). • Teen children found it less enjoyable.

Mobile Applications and Internet-based Approaches for Supporting Non-professional Caregivers

Pediatric population Study design Sample size	Description of the Intervention	Results	Findings on usability of technology
Atopic dermatitis RCT CGs of 98 children. Only 73 completed the study (37 intervention & 36 control) (post-intervention questionnaire) Bergmo, 2009[48]	Software that allowed secure messaging. Parents sent photos of child's eczema, with written description to the specialist. Also, they could fill in a form about the problem and the symptoms. The specialist responded with treatment advice. Control group used traditional means for dermatology care.	• Intervention patients had fewer visits to providers of complementary medicine than controls, mean difference=0.8 vs. 0.09, $F_{(1,66)}=2.96$ (P=0.09). • No change in self management behavior. No change in health outcomes. No change in costs for parents.	• Showed the feasibility of doing consults via secure message, but did not show improved outcomes. • 79% of users would recommend its use to others.
Cancer RCT 104 mothers randomized to Problem-Solving Skills Training (PSST) and 93 to the PSST+Personal Digital Assistant (PDA) arm Askins, 2009[49]	Randomized trial comparing traditional PSST versus PSST+PDA reminder device. PDA did four things: 1) review problem-solving process; 2) review and practice the five elements of the problem-solving approach; 3) prompt the user to use the problem-solving skills; and 4) daily log to record problems confronted by the mother.	No differences were found on the outcome measures between the traditional PSST group and the PSST+PDA on problem-solving skills, improved mood, reduction of depressive symptoms, and reduction of PTSD symptoms.	• Mothers in PSST+PDA group had lower willingness to recommend their program than those in the PSST alone group, 7.8 (1.9) vs. 8.6 (0.92), P<0.01. • Among PDA users, 55% thought they were easy to keep (e.g. store and carry). Almost all said they were comfortable with text size, wording, and volume of the audio-recorder feature. • 71% said the information in the program was organized and understandable. Entering text and audio was seen as helpful, but use of voice recorder was problematic. • The computer-animated character ("Gina") was seen as helpful, providing directions for using the computer program, applying the problem-solving process, and helping participants "feel better". 60% liked working with Gina, and 49% said Gina understood their problems • There were substantial difficulties in transferring data from the PDAs to the computers, making some analyses impossible.
Cancer, newly diagnosed Usability study using a survey and interview 21 families Ewing, 2009[50]	Web site with multiple features: a) home page; b) information and exercises for coping; c) five discussion groups for different age groups; d) Ask an Expert feature; e) Q&A library; f) Resources: links to other relevant websites and local Pittsburgh resources. Usability was assessed using a 9-item version of the Website Evaluation Instrument (WEI). Qualitative interviews were conducted after the study with 24 caregivers (including from families that did and did not access the website).	• Eleven individuals from 9 of the 21 families logged on to the website; five of these were caregivers, 4 were cancer patients, and 2 were siblings of the patients. • Most commonly used sections were Discussion Groups (n=257 hits); Common Areas of Concern (n=78 hits); Previously Asked Questions (n=66 hits); and Connect to Coping (n=60 hits). • Nonuse of the web site was related to dislike/unfamiliarity of computers (24%) and being too busy (21%). • Other reasons given for not using the website (not quantified) were spending time in hospitals where no Internet; already having sufficient information from research and medical staff, and preferring face-to-face interactions instead of computer discussion groups. • Among the 5 caregivers who accessed the website, most helpful aspects were "Ask the Expert" and "Previously Asked Questions". • Caregivers believed their children did not use the website because they wanted to feel "normal," had sufficient support from family and friends; were too sick; or only used computer for talking to friends. • Hands-on training (as opposed to phone training) appeared to be associated with greater use of the tool.	Not discussed. Relatively low use may have been related to this being a high stress time for the families (i.e. shortly after diagnosis of the child with cancer). The participants may have been too tired and overwhelmed to be able to use this site.

Mobile Applications and Internet-based Approaches for Supporting Non-professional Caregivers

Pediatric population Study design Sample size	Description of the Intervention	Results	Findings on usability of technology
Cancer Survey 73 parents Han, 2001[51]	No Intervention. Evaluation study of 3 on-line support groups (cancer-N-BASTOMA, n=17 parents participated; PED-ALL, n=28 parents participated; and PED-ONC, n=28 parents) of parents of children with cancer. Participants received a survey, with structured and open-ended questions, about the use of computers for support.	• Most (85%) connected daily to the group, while 11% connected 1 to 3 times a week. • Mean time connected to the computer group was 5 hours (SD=6.1), with range of 30 min. to 40 hours. • Most commonly cited advantage was information giving and receiving (cited by 77%), followed by sharing experiences (e.g. gives a sense they are not alone) (67%), general support (29%), venting feelings (14%), accessibility (8%), and use of text (3%). • Disadvantages included noise (i.e. off topic messages) (49%), negative emotions (e.g. when you hear bad news from others)(26%), large volume of mail (21%), and lack of physical face-to-face contact (11%).	• Technically feasible. • The online support group appeared to provide emotional and interpersonal support to caregivers, though some users were overwhelmed by the sheer volume of posts/messages, and number of irrelevant/off topic posts.
Cancer Observational study 12 families Lewis, 2006[52]	Caring Connection is a web-portal to improve family to provider and family to family communication. Includes email, access to laboratory data, current medication lists. (This appears to be a kind of personal health record designed for the caregiver.)	• Caregivers used the system an average of 1-2 times a day • Greater use appears to occur in the period shortly after diagnosis. • Qualitative data indicate caregivers like access to laboratory data; also of interest is medication lists.	• Caregivers appeared to appreciate greater access to information that typically was only available in paper medical record; easy access to labs results and medication lists was appreciated.
Cerebral palsy Observational study, Holland 30 parents and 120 health professionals Gulmans, 2010[53]	System allows parents to communicate (i.e. a kind of messaging system) with health providers (wide range of professionals). Also enables professionals to communicate with each other.	• 43% of parents compared to 14% of professionals used the system. • Parents submitted a mean of 5 questions (range 1-17) and 3 responses (range 1-9). Professionals submitted a mean of 2 questions (range 1-8) and 4 responses (range 1-23). Purpose of the submitted questions was for consultation or advice, information sharing, monitoring, and administrative purposes. • The rehabilitation physician was most often the person identified as responsible for feedback (41% of the 111 submitted questions), followed by physiotherapist (20%) occupational therapist (14%); teacher/supervisor (10%). • Of the 21 parents who used the system, 40% used it regularly, 50% occasionally, and 10% rarely. • Nearly all parents (95%) found it valuable (all but one). They liked the accessibility (access 24-7); efficiency (avoid frustrating phone calls); and the transparency. • Professionals use the system substantially less than parents and used it less often. Only 29% of professional found it valuable.	• Parents and professionals thought usability/ease of use could be better, e.g. by simplifying the log-in procedure. • Some parents proposed linking the system to an online support group. • May work best with parents who have complex network of providers and organizations that they need to interact with.

Mobile Applications and Internet-based Approaches for Supporting Non-professional Caregivers

Pediatric population Study design Sample size	Description of the Intervention	Results	Findings on usability of technology
Cystic fibrosis, diabetes or arthritis Usability study with satisfaction questionnaire 16 parents Britto, 2009[54]	Prototype pediatric portal with test data. Participants were given scenario-based usability testing tasks. Measures included time to complete tasks; videotaping while using "think aloud" technique, followed by content analysis; Computer Usability Satisfaction Questionnaire (CUSQ).	• Caregivers liked assistance dealing with insurance companies, and preparing for the doctor's visit. • Problems identified were use of medical jargon such as the abbreviation "Fe" or what a pathology report was. • Other challenges were figuring how to interpret graphs, and understanding laboratory results that had abbreviations and values. • They asked for fewer clicks to find things; some wanted more medication information such as side effects and allergy issues. • For email, they wanted some kind of confirmation that it was received by a provider.	• Researchers found several areas where usability could be improved including finding date of last pulmonary function test was completed by only one person. • Finding and interpreting lab results was also a challenge; but improvements to the system made it easier to find in Round 3. • Sending email was also challenging but improved as the system improved. • Satisfaction was about the same regardless of the round of testing.
Dental RCT 158 in the text message group, 160 controls Nelson, 2011[55]	Computer-generated text message to cell phone of parent/caregiver 48 hours before the child's appointment. Controls received voice reminders on cell phone.	No-show rates were lower in the control group (voice reminder on cell phone)(8.2%) compared to the intervention group (text message reminder) (17.7%), p=0.011.	• Not formally tested. • Authors hypothesize that the text messages may be perceived as impersonal, whereas the voice reminders were from staff that many of the patients would know personally. • Currently VA does not consider text messages a secure means of communication. If it were simply for appointment reminders, this might be acceptable.
Depression Usability study involving qualitative interviews of 33 CGs of youth who had been psychiatrically hospitalized Demaso, 2006[56]	A web-based application for caregiver to share personal stories about caring for their child with depression. Includes writings of experiences, poems, stories, video clips. It is designed to encourage and facilitate networking and social support among a community of caregivers.	• Satisfaction with tool high (mean 5.75 (SD 1.66) on 7 pt scale). • Satisfied with way stories presented, 6.19 (0.95). • Satisfied with factual information, 5.44 (1.70). • Rating of hurtfulness, 1.43 (1.14). • Potential harm to youth, 1.79 (1.14). • No negative impact on relationship with child. • 8 parents thought there were parts that were not helpful. This related to repetitive factual information, or material that may not be appropriate for the website, i.e. bipolar, and medications issues. • 18 said parent stories most helpful. 14 said youth stories most helpful. • 3 subjects said parts were hurtful, including "sadness and worry" realizing child was depressed; and "hurtfulness" learning how many youth are depressed. • Ideas for improvement included greater number and range of stories, i.e. beyond hospitalization stage (n=3), geared to younger audience (n=2); more info on meds (n=2) and narratives by siblings and extended family members (n=2). • Other suggestions were for more info on meds (n=2), more specific advice for parents (n=2), and more information on community resources (n=2). Two suggestions to make the web site more interactive, e.g. Q&A forum with providers, and parent-to-parent forum. • Specific impacts were highest for giving a sense that others are dealing with same issues (mean=6.44 (SD=0.91) on 7 pt scale), helpful to read about other families, 6.06 (1.39), decreases isolation 5.83 (1.51), increases hope, 5.44 (1.42) increases their understanding of the experience, 5,4 (1.38) and increase sense of perspective, 5.26 (1.56).	Was not assessed in a systematic way. Social networking reduces sense of isolation; however, 8 parents thought there were parts of the website that were not helpful. This related to repetitive factual information, or material that may not be appropriate for the website, i.e. bipolar and medications issues.

Mobile Applications and Internet-based Approaches for Supporting Non-professional Caregivers Evidence-based Synthesis Program

Pediatric population Study design Sample size	Description of the Intervention	Results	Findings on usability of technology
		• Coping: 29 said it helped understand symptoms of depression, 24 said it gave sense of how common depression is, 19 said it increased their understanding of their child's experience. • Attitude change: there was a moderate degree of attitude change (did the tool help you understand your and your family's feelings about childhood depression, mean 4.88 (SD not provided); do you think the tool had any effect on how supportive you and your family are of each other, mean 3.41 (SD not provided)).	
Diabetes Key informant interviews (n=9) and technology feedback questionnaire (n=10) subsequent to an RCT (n=22) Keshavjee, 2003[57]	PDA tool designed to improve communication between caregivers and patients. RCT was stopped early because PDA intervention did not meet functionality expectations.	None reported.	Low usability: interviews and questionnaires revealed multiple points of failure including lack of patient/parent time or energy to use device, malfunction of glucometer, lack of connectivity with an ISP (especially an issue for rural participants).
Diabetes Usability survey 23 respondents (16 mothers, 3 fathers, 4 teenage patients) Nordfeldt, 2010[58]	Web portal with multiple functionalities including diabetes-related information, social networking, online simulation software, prescription renewal, appointment scheduling, contact information.	• Perceived reliability of content was important (local practitioners were responsible for portal content). • Perception that information is outdated or used infrequently could lead to decline in use over time. • Users can generate useful information to share with others, but this utility is likely to be weakened by low traffic on site. • Login requirement to access site limited its use. Most common negative experiences with portal were access related issues.	• Feasible, but upkeep would require resources. • In order to be perceived as useful, CHIT needs to be updated frequently and have a certain critical mass of users (if there is a social networking component). Also, the login access issues seem an important barrier as well.
Influenza RCT of 7,547 children who had not received prior flu vaccine 3,790 randomized to intervention, 3,784 to usual care Stockwell, 2012[59]	Parents received up to 5 weekly text messages. Messaging system was linked to an immunization registry. The messages included educational information about the vaccine, and information about Saturday flu vaccine clinics. Texts were personalized (e.g. had child's name in body of text).	Higher proportion of intervention group received immunization, compared to controls. 42.6% of intervention (n=1653) compared to usual care (39.9%; n=1509) had received flu vaccine as of March 31, 2011, (difference=3.7%; CI=1.5%-5.9%), relative rate ratio=1.09 (1.04-1.15; P=0.001). At the earlier (fall 2010) review date the difference also existed: 27.1%,n=1026 vs. 22.8%,n=864 (difference=4.3%; CI=2.3%-6.3%), RRR=1.19 (1.10-1.28; P<0.001).	• Low income populations that are traditionally hard to reach were responsive to text messaging technology for preventive care reminders. • Currently VA discourages text messages for clinical care because they are not felt to be secure. • Feasible; might initially need a vendor the does large scale texting.
Liver transplant Pre-post study 41 patients, mean age 15 (range 2-27) Miloh, 2009[60]	Automated text messaging system. Participants logged in on line and entered name/contact info for patient and caregiver, medication name and frequency, and desired time for alerts. Messages initially sent to person responsible for medication administration (patient or caregiver). If they did not send back message confirming med intake, caregiver would be notified after 30 mins elapsed.	Outcomes included tacrolimus level SD (higher the SD, higher risk of rejection), and biopsy-proven rejection episodes. Mean tacrolimus SD: Pre: 3.46 µg/L, Post: 1.37 µg/L (P <.005) Biopsy-proven rejection in one year (data available for all 41 pts) - Pre: 12/41, Post: 2/41, (P = 0.02).	• High attrition (37%). • Simple, potentially feasible intervention that could potentially be useful for adult transplant patients (or similar disease dependent on strict adherence).

Mobile Applications and Internet-based Approaches for Supporting Non-professional Caregivers

Pediatric population Study design Sample size	Description of the Intervention	Results	Findings on usability of technology
Neonatal ICU Retrospective cohort study across 4 hospitals 81 records available of 135 (drop outs included deaths, transfers and 27 whose parents never used the program) Safran, 2005[61]	Baby CareLink includes multiple functions - parents receive daily updates from NICU, see recent pics of baby, communicate with NICU staff, access personalized knowledge base for newborn care, provide feedback re: care process. Nurses could communicate with parents via the portal. Access to medical reference library also available. Post d/c, the program also used to support care coordination and follow-up coordination.	• LOS comparing parents who viewed < 3 pages/d to those who viewed ≥ 3 pages/d: reduction in LOS among high use group compared to low use group was 17.5 days, p = 0.03.	Apparently, company no longer in existence.
Post-ER visit Uncontrolled trial N=303 parents Goldman, 2005[62]	Final culture results (positive and negative) were posted on a website for parents to access. An email was sent to the parent telling them the culture result was available on the website.	• 61% (186/303) accessed their child's culture result on the Internet system. • Eighty percent (243/303) of families were reached for follow-up and 27% of these (66/243) reported they had "no time" to go to the website to view results, 10% had lost their login ID, and 20% did not use for other reasons; 43% (104/243) of those reached for follow-up accessed the system within 5 days after results were posted and before receiving a phone call from the research assistant. • The time from sending the email notifying the family that results were posted until the results had been viewed was mean of 94 hours (range 1 minute to 611 hours). • Of 141 families (104 at 5-day follow-up, plus 37 at 10-day follow-up) who retrieved information from website and who were reached for follow-up, 16% printed the information, 26% reported the results to a family physician or pediatrician, and 5% had changes in treatment made because of the results they saw on the website.	• About 10 to 12% reported that they lost the ID number that would allow them to get the culture results. • Training could have helped to reduce the numbers of parents who never accessed the system. • This study points to the feasibility and interest from caregivers of having access to cultures/lab results of the family member they are caring for. Majority of parents seemed to appreciate the opportunity to find the culture results online. This kind of access is now built into most electronic Personal Health Record systems.
Sleep disturbance RCT 264 mothers and their infants/toddlers Mindell, 2011[63]	The Customized Sleep Profile (CSP) program provides parents with individualized information (based on parent survey responses) in three domains: 1) normative comparison of their child to other children, on sleep patterns; 2) rating of their child as excellent, good, or disrupted sleeper; 3) customized advice on how to help their child sleep better. Study had 3 arms: a) algorithmic Internet-based intervention; b) algorithmic Internet intervention PLUS prescribed bedtime routine; c) control group.	• Maternal sleep improved (onset latency, total sleep time, number and duration of night wakings, sleep efficiency, total sleep quality) P<0.001; at end of treatment, 25% of mothers in control group were good sleepers vs. 33.3% in Internet group and 47.6% in Internet + routine group (Chi-sq=10.72; p=0.005). • Maternal mood improved, measured by Profile of Mood States (POMS). Significant improvements for mothers in the Internet + routine group were found for all subscales of the POMS (P < 0.001). For mothers in the Internet only group, there were significant improvements in tension, depression, fatigue, and confusion (P < 0.001). • Overall, children in intervention groups had decreased sleep onset latency, decreased number/duration of night wakings, increased sleep continuity, and increased nighttime sleep (P < 0.001). Examples: for Internet group number of night wakings went from 1.81 to 1.44 to 0.99, from baseline, to week 2, to week 3 (p<.001), whereas no significant difference for the control group. There were few significant differences found for the control group.	• Tailored sleep instruction for parents of children was very helpful in the short-term in reducing child sleep difficulties and improving mood of mothers. • Survey responses indicated satisfaction with the intervention, i.e. 90% found the recommendations helpful; and 93% stating they would continue to use recommendations after the study. • Usability testing not well described but it appears that it was assessed by a small number of survey items.

Mobile Applications and Internet-based Approaches for Supporting Non-professional Caregivers

Pediatric population Study design Sample size	Description of the Intervention	Results	Findings on usability of technology
TBI RCT, 26 families allocated to OFPS, 20 to IRC Wade, 2006[64] Post-hoc analysis of RCT compared 14 parents with prior computer experience to 6 parents with no experience Carey, 2008[65] Observational study of 19 participants in 6 families Wade, 2004[66]	The web component of the Online Family Problem-Solving (OFPS) includes logistic information and educational material which is presented in 12-14 separate sessions. There are core sessions and optional sessions assigned based on family need. Sessions were interactive, with families entering responses to questions and receiving feedback from Web site. Exercises completed by family stored and reviewed by a therapist. Each session paired with a synchronous on-line videoconferencing session with therapist. Control group received IRC which consisted of access to static TBI information on Web. All families in both groups received necessary computing equipment.	• Parents with no history of prior computer use were less likely to benefit from OFPS intervention (see Wade studies). The improvements in depression and anxiety seen with OFPS were limited to those parents who had prior experience with computers. • Depression (CES-D): OFPS v IRC, mean (SD) 9.25 (7.09) v 18.15 (13.49), p <.05 • Anxiety inventory: OFPS v IRC, mean (SD) 9.25 (4.99) v 14.05 (7.50), p <.05 • Global psychiatric symptoms (SCL-90-R): OFPS v IRC, mean (SD) 73.45 (9.61) v 69.16 (10.02), p >.05 • Analysis of moderators of treatment efficacy found only parental socioeconomic status and social advantage were correlated with caregiver outcomes. • Effects of OFPS did not appear to be entirely mediated through changes in parental problem solving skills.[64]	• Feasible but quite resource intensive: each family was given a computer, printer, and webcam for the intervention, and in-person training on use of equipment/intervention done by an RA. • Parents with no prior computer experience were more likely to miss sessions. • Families ranked web site as moderately to very easy to use. • The type of webcam affected favorability ratings of the videoconferencing as did the audio interface. • Half of the computers were infected with viruses. • All but 1 parent rated Web site as moderately to extremely easy to use.[64] • The study population was not highly educated (about half had no more than high school education), suggesting a complex web-based intervention may be feasible in populations with varied educational backgrounds.[64]
TBI Observational study of 9 families with teens with TBI. RCT of same 9 families comparing TOPS with and without audio. Wade, 2008[67,68]	Teen Online Problem Solving Intervention (TOPS). Similar to the OFPS described above, but some of the specific content was different and focused more on executive function skills.	• TOPS intervention reduced parental depression and distress, and improved communication between parents and children. • Conflict Behavior Questionnaire (CBQ - measures parent-adolescent communication), pre v post scores: 4.58 (4.40) v 2.08 (1.78), p = 0.04 • Global psychiatric symptoms (SCL-90-R), pre v post scores: 53.00 (12.66) v 50.83 (10.51), p = 0.30 • CES-D, pre v post scores: 13.17 (9.11) v 6.92 (6.36), p =.01 • Child Behavior Checklist (CBCL - parent reported measure of child behavior problems): fewer internalizing symptoms post-intervention, no difference in total score • Children's Depression Inventory (CDI), pre and post scores: 1.56 (1.51) v 0.67 (0.71), p = 0.02	• All families completed all modules.[67] • Most participants found website very or extremely easy to use. • Almost all participants agreed they reached goals they had for program. • All families completed all 10 core sessions. Average time spent on each session: 40 min.[68]
Traumatic injury excluding TBI. Pre-post study comparing 25 parents who received the interactive web intervention to 25 who received only a DVD of the educational video segments Marsac, 2011[69]	Educational video segments, parents can rate specific child reactions and receive tailored tips in a care plan.	• Parents reported high levels of satisfaction with web site and with video intervention. • Interactive web group more likely report they would use intervention tools in the future than video only group (76 vs 44%, p < 0.05). • Otherwise, no real differences between video and interactive web groups.	• Not formally assessed. • Interactive web intervention did not seem to produce different knowledge or satisfaction results than video-only intervention, though sample was small and baseline knowledge among this well-educated sample was high.

KEY QUESTION #3. What are the major gaps in the consumer health information technology literature serving non-professional caregivers of adult patients with regards to technology development, availability, and/or evaluation?

Table 3 summarizes the interactive applications and functionality of the interventions included in this review, and indicates the current phase of the interventions' lifecycle at the time of publication.

The CHIT literature reflects a relatively new, developing field. Most studies described interventions in early development (ten studies) or pilot-tested (five studies) on a small scale. Only seven studies were developed to evaluate health outcomes, but most of these were relatively small studies. There is a dearth of literature describing the health outcome effects of CHIT in larger populations. Some of the larger studies involved interventions, such as text messaging, which might be logistically simpler to deploy and test on a large scale. Almost no studies evaluated the actual implementation of interventions that had already been tested and found to be efficacious.

Reviewed studies were also not designed to qualitatively develop a contextual understanding of the use of the intervention technology. At this time, there is not information to assess how these interventions fit into the day-to-day lives of caregivers. Additionally, there is relatively little information about how caregiver demographic characteristics affect the user experience. These are promising areas for future research; however, longer horizons will be necessary to assess usage over time given that caregivers' needs for information, skills, and support are likely to evolve.

Intervention content varied widely. Nearly half the interventions, interestingly, included a component designed to facilitate peer communication. On the other hand, despite the focus on supporting caregivers, relatively few interventions included components specifically designed to enhance communication between caregivers and patients. Similarly few studies analyzed outcomes separately for caregiver and patient users; notable exceptions were CHESS,[23] Caring~Web,[27] WECARE,[34] and The Schizophrenia Guide.[35] Thus, it largely remains unclear if there are differences between caregivers and patients in their interactions with and benefit derived from technology. This likely has implications for perceptions of value, usability, utility, and satisfaction, as well as usage and challenges to adoption. Studies that simultaneously enroll both the patient and caregiver as a dyad, as was performed in CHESS,[23] WECARE,[34] and Dew et al.[38] may provide an opportunity to better understand these relationships. The question of whether technology implementations should be designed for the caregiver or the patient, or both as the end user is not answerable from the current literature, and may be best addressed by expert opinion and consensus. Other important gaps include an understanding of how these mobile interventions complement existing services. We also found very little information about the cost-effectiveness of CHIT.

Table 3. Summary of the functionalities available in health informatics interventions to support non-professional caregivers, stratified by care-recipient population

Study	Reminders, Notification	Education Modules, Build skills	Self-Care, Feedback	Peer-Peer	Caregiver-Patient	Caregiver-Professional	Transaction Tool	Development	Pilot	Evaluation
Alzheimer's and cognitive impairment										
Alzheimer's Caregiver Internet Support System (ACISS) Vehvilainen, 2002[14]		√		√		√			√	
AlzOnline Glueckauf, 2004[71]		√		√		√				√
Becker, 2006[15]	√		√					√		
Caregiver's Friend: Dealing with Dementia Beauchamp, 2005[16]		√				√				√
Internet-based support services (ICSS) for Chinese caregivers of people with AD Chiu, 2005[17] Chiu, 2009[18]						√			√	
ComputerLink Bass, 1998[19] Brennan, 1995[20]		√		√		√				√
Network Interaction Therapy Kuwahara, 2004[21]			√		√			√		
Cancer										
OncoLife Hill-Kayser, 2009[22]			√					√		
Comprehensive Health Enhancement Support System (CHESS) Namkoong, 2011[23]		√	√	√		√				√
Nolan, 2006[24]				√						√
Prostate Interactive Education System (PIES) Diefenbach, 2004[25]			√					√		
Stroke										
Caring~Web Pierce, 2009[26] Steiner, 2008[27]		√		√		√				√
Mental illness or traumatic brain injury										
Stjernsward, 2011[32]			√	√				√		
Glynn, 2010[33]		√		√		√		√		

Study	Intervention Application/Functionality Category							Phase in Intervention Lifecycle		
	Reminders, Notification	Education Modules, Build skills	Self-Care, Feedback	Peer-Peer	Caregiver-Patient	Caregiver-Professional	Transaction Tool	Development	Pilot	Evaluation
Web Enabled Caregiver Access to Resources and Education (WE CARE) Rotondi, 2005[34]		√		√		√		√		
The Schizophrenia Guide Rotondi, 2005[35]		√		√		√			√	
Chiu, 2006[36]			√		√			√		
Surgery and heart transplantation										
Huang, 2006[37]	√							√		
Dew, 2004[38]		√		√		√				√
Frail elderly, disabled NOS, and home parenteral nutrition										
Assisting Carers using Telematics Interventions to meet Older Persons' Needs (ACTION) Magnusson, 2005[40] Chambers, 2002[39] Magnusson, 2005[41]		√	√	√		√			√	
Finn, 1999[42]				√				√		
HPN Family Caregivers Website Fitzgerald, 2011[43]		√	√						√	
Studies in pediatric populations										
ADHD Ossebaard, 2010[44]		√						√		
Arthritis Stinson, 2010[45]		√	√	√				√		
Asthma Krishna, 2000[46] Krishna, 2003[47]		√								√
Atopic dermatitis Bergmo, 2009[48]						√				√
Cancer Askins, 2009[49]		√	√							√
Cancer Ewing, 2009[50]		√		√		√		√		
Cancer Han, 2001[51]				√				√		
Cancer: Caring Connection[52]				√	√			√		
Cerebral palsy Gulmans, 2010[53]						√		√		

Study	Intervention Application/Functionality Category							Phase in Intervention Lifecycle		
	Reminders, Notification	Education Modules, Build skills	Self-Care, Feedback	Peer-Peer	Caregiver-Patient	Caregiver-Professional	Transaction Tool	Development	Pilot	Evaluation
Cystic fibrosis, diabetes, or arthritis Britto, 2009[54]			√			√		√		
Dental Nelson, 2011[55]	√									√
Depression Demaso, 2006[56]				√				√		
Diabetes Keshavjee, 2003[57]			Unclear					√		
Diabetes Nordfeldt, 2010[58]		√	√	√		√	√	√		
Influenza Stockwell, 2012[59]	√									√
Liver transplant Miloh, 2009[60]	√									√
Neonatal ICU: Baby CareLink Safran, 2005[61]		√	√			√				√
Post-ER visit Goldman, 2005[62]	√								√	
Sleep disturbance: Customized Sleep Profile (CSP) Mindell, 2011[63]			√							√
TBI: Online Family Problem-Solving (OFPS) Carey, 2008[65] Wade, 2004[66] Wade, 2006[64]		√				√				√
TBI: Teen Online Problem Solving Intervention (TOPS) Wade, 2008[67] Wade, 2009[68]		√				√			√	
Traumatic injury excluding TBI Marsac, 2011[69]		√	√						√	

DISCUSSION

As the need for most cost-effective and resource-limited healthcare services gains greater urgency, the VA plans to expand CHIT web and mobile applications for patients and caregivers is essential. A small but growing body of literature examines CHIT interventions developed and tested for non-professional caregivers. Overall, a broad diversity of interventions has been identified; the majority were multi-component online tools intended to improve knowledge, skills and coping, and provide social support of caregivers. Many of these interventions offered communication functions such as online peer support groups, email access to clinicians such as nurse specialists, and educational content promoting stress-relief, wellbeing, and coping skills.

Studies also reported a broad diversity of outcomes with little consistency, including patient-centered outcomes, usability, usage, and user-perceptions. The one exception being that user satisfaction was frequently reported. In all, only six studies in seven publications reported caregiver burden, strain or other caregiver-centered outcomes in the adult literature.[16,18,20,23,26,38] Given the heterogeneity of interventions and measured outcomes, as well as of the evaluative methodologies used, it is difficult to draw over-arching conclusions regarding the impact of these technologies on caregivers, patients, or health systems.

Common intervention components

Online support groups were common among the interventions, and often the most frequently used component. Online support groups were typically threaded discussions on the website or group emails that facilitated asynchronous communication. Only one intervention provided real-time, *synchronous* communication in an online chat room so that multiple family members of a schizophrenic patient could participate in an online, professionally-mediated group therapy session despite the family members being in disparate locations.[33] *Asynchronous*, online support groups have advantages compared to their in-person counterparts such as mitigating obstacles of distance and time-constraints, as discussed previously.

Formal online support groups with restricted membership enrollments that are organized around specific applications and interventions may have benefits not seen in the *informal, loosely structured*, Internet interest groups, message boards, and chat rooms more typically seen on the web.[23] CHESS investigators suggested that while the latter builds community around a shared condition or illness, formal online support group participants experience an increased sense of belonging as a result of restricted group membership, association with a single institution or organization, linked educational components, and shared clinical providers. Multiple studies also speculated on the benefits of professionally-mediated online discussions.[27,28,32,33,38] Usually, the participating professional was a nurse specialist prompting discussion with thought-provoking questions or providing a clinical perspective to the online support group. Finn et al. believed that such a curator role was essential to re-direct misinformation.[42] Rotondi et al. suggested that a curator may be necessary to quell negative comments, although in their experience, such events were rare.[34] The benefits and unintended consequences of a moderator within a peer support function persist as an issue.

Applications allowing users to pose questions to a clinician were frequently included in the interventions. In the adult literature, interventions provided this functionality via an email to a nurse specialist from the website; none used alternative technology such as SMS/text messaging or web-based forms. In the pediatrics literature, use of SMS/text messaging in the evaluated intervention was quite common. A possible explanation is that parents in the pediatric literature are likely younger on average than their counterparts who are caring for adults with chronic illnesses. Thus, parents of young children and adolescents may be more familiar with current mobile phone and computing technologies. Regardless, caregivers appreciated the access to clinicians both through mediated online discussion groups and email "Ask an Expert" functions as it increased their perceptions of support and self-confidence.[73]

Providing distinct, parallel, private online support groups each for caregivers and patients – that was inaccessible to the other – was emphasized by two studies.[34,38] Caregivers in particular held that they were "better able to voice their concerns in a separate forum" and that this was crucial to promote candid, reflective online discussions.

Generalizability

Many studies may reflect utility in highly selected populations. Most studies do not report details regarding the recruitment process, thus it remains unknown how many potential-users did not sign-up for the study, and how they might differ from the study population. For example, the only adult study reporting this data found that as many as 45 percent of those approached declined to sign-up because they were too busy, under too much stress, or did not see utility in the intervention.[18]

Several studies questioned whether Internet-based applications are appropriate for all users. Concerns include a lack of human contact in online communications;[28] online support groups may not provide the equivalent emotional support of in-person groups;[34] caregivers may not welcome outside, non-familial support;[30] caregivers may reject technology-based support because it is too costly, of insufficient quality, or not geared to their routines and preferences; and replacement of face-to-face interactions with Internet applications may not be appropriate for caregivers who are particularly overstretched and overburdened, as such individuals may require more active support than can be provided online.[41] Some of the most highly valued components, such as online support groups, might have less benefit in younger populations that are already comfortable with using existing social networking applications, such as Facebook.

Some studies included accommodations specifically meant to increase intervention applicability for older caregiver populations,[15,41] but many studies reported on caregiver users with a mean age of 55 to 60 years. Magnusson et al. corrected a common misconception in their assertion that the elderly are not inherently negative about technology but, instead, require additional training and learning time, and increased computer/Internet access and support compared to younger users.[73] Older caregivers may also benefit from applications with special accommodations for aging vision and manual dexterity.

The applicability and transferability of the interventions to a VA population remain unclear as only one study specifically evaluated Veterans. Many of the interventions could conceivably be applicable to caregivers of Veterans. For example, a number of interventions targeted conditions frequently seen in Veteran populations such as dementia, cancer, and traumatic brain injury.

While several studies detailed their security procedures,[17,18,32,33,35] many studies provided relatively little information. Whether these procedures meet VA's standards for privacy and information security would need to be determined. However, no studies reported privacy concerns from a patient or caregiver perspective.

Additional barriers to technology implementation

Some investigators raised specific concerns about incorporating Internet technologies in to the collection of care services already being provided. Among these were that users will still have time constraints that may preclude taking full advantage of online resources,[23] the challenges of designing tailored resources for a broad diversity of users with different cultural backgrounds,[34] complications of medical practice when users/patients may reside in neighboring states in which their providers are not licensed,[35] and systems to adequately manage emergencies that are revealed online (such as suicidality).[33]

User experience

Technology development infrequently involves the end user, often resulting in underutilization or rejection of the intervention.[41] Many investigators asserted that patients and caregivers should be included in development of intervention content, not just to ensure harmonization with the caregivers' current life process and perception of need,[30] but also to "validate and reinforce the importance of their role."[41] Several researchers described qualitative, observational data regarding the types of content that caregivers desired. Keaton et al. state that adults learn experientially, and need information that is immediately useful and relevant to their situation.[28] Pierce et al. found that caregivers wanted additional information about the care-recipients' medical conditions.[31] Rotondi et al. described their unpublished data suggesting caregivers want better skills for dealing with the medical, cognitive, and behavioral sequelae of illness and injuries, and assistance identifying additional community and financial resources.

Formal usability testing was seldom described in the literature; however, tools do exist, including the Website Analysis and Measurement Inventory (WAMMI)[39] and System Usability Score (SUS).[32] In addition, a U.S. government website provides other tools for measuring usability, as well as descriptions of underlying principles.[77]

Inability of users to access website content was frequently acknowledged in studies. In some cases, these issues could not be overcome despite provision of computers, Internet connectivity and/or training to users. Familiarity and comfort with technology was cited as a possible explanation, which may disproportionately affect older adults. Magnusson et al. asserted that the elderly are not inherently negative about technology but have increased challenges due to less computer access, requiring longer training, and a lack of confidence.[73] Additional allowances for training and education may overcome such barriers, and technology can accommodate for the physical deterioration of age or chronic illness such as decreased vision and mobility.

Three pediatric studies raised potential concerns regarding online support groups. Parents of children with cancer experienced distress to postings about the death of a child.[51] Two other studies cited the need for a critical mass of participants to foster active discussion.[32,50]

LIMITATIONS

In setting out to perform a systematic review of a new healthcare technology, a chief limitation is the pace of change. The healthcare mobile application market is seeing unprecedented growth and dissemination. Although research is ongoing, the evidence base within the published literature has yet to appear. Thus, while this was intended to be an expansive review, we noted that many relatively new technologies such as text-messaging, tweeting, and interactive, game-based applications were not represented in the articles captured and reviewed.

Our review focused on CHIT used by caregivers; we acknowledge there are technologies tested only in patients that could conceivably be used by caregivers, but these were outside of the scope of this review. Of note, our review scope also excluded telehealth and telemedicine interventions, even though these are interventions that could potentially be adapted to mobile platforms – these are the subject of other reviews.[78-81] The review also excluded interactive voice response, or IVR, technology. IVR systems are automated, computerized telephonic interventions that deliver individualized messages and collect feedback from targeted users through voice recognition and telephone keypads. Though outside the scope of our review, IVR has promise as a CHIT intervention, particularly in populations with lower access to the Internet or smartphones or for delivering less complex interventions. IVR has been assessed in a variety of settings and medical conditions relevant to VA, including depression,[82] tobacco use,[83] post-discharge care,[84] heart failure and diabetes.[85] IVR appears acceptable to patients including those with mental health conditions,[85] and has shown positive effects on patient behavior related to screening, prevention, treatment follow-up and medication reminders.[86,87]

The lack of a common taxonomy for CHIT might have made it more difficult to find all potentially relevant intervention studies as they may have been indexed in ways that we did not cover in our search strategy. We used a broad search strategy (Appendix A), and we searched bibliographies of included articles. Finally, as this is primarily an exploratory review, we did not conduct formal quality assessment of included studies. Many of the included studies represented pilot or developmental phase interventions with numerous methodologic weaknesses such as lack of control groups and small sample sizes. The results of this review should not be interpreted to provide definitive evidence about intervention efficacy.

CONCLUSION

There is a growing literature of CHIT interventions that are being developed for non-professional caregivers. Overall, a broad diversity of interventions has been identified; the majority were multi-component online tools intended to improve knowledge, skills and coping, and provide social support of caregivers. Many of these interventions offered communication functions such as online peer support groups; email access to clinicians such as nurse specialists; and educational content promoting stress-relief, wellbeing, and coping skills. However, usability testing was infrequently reported. Given the heterogeneity of interventions and measured outcomes, as well as of the evaluative methodologies used, it is difficult to draw over-arching conclusions regarding the impact of these technologies on caregiver, patient, or health system outcomes. Formal usability testing can identify important challenges and should be incorporated more often in the development process. Patients and caregivers should be involved in the design and improvement of interventions.

Below is a list that summarizes the emerging themes and future research directions for CHIT interventions:

- Consumer health technologies for caregivers may improve caregiver strain, coping strategies, self-efficacy, intention to obtain additional support, depression, anxiety, and anger.
- Online access to expert care from healthcare providers via text-messing, Q&A, FAQs, etc. are also highly valued and may supplement existing communications.
- Text-messaging systems can reach significant numbers of caregivers and have been examined as a way to enhance compliance to medications and preventive health actions.
- The asynchronous nature of communication in online peer support groups and text-messaging may facilitate participation by mitigating geographic and temporal barriers.
- Online peer support groups and chat rooms were the most-used and most-valued components in several interventions.
- In online support groups, anonymity through the use of a Screen Name or User ID was valued by caregivers and patients, and should be incorporated.
- Privacy issues did not emerge as a major concern for caregivers and patients and should not necessarily be perceived as a barrier to the development of consumer health technologies.
- Technical barriers and lack of familiarity with technology are the most frequently cited reasons for failure to participate in a technology intervention.

Future directions:

- Consumer health technologies may reduce the frequency of emergency visits and hospitalizations.
- Benefits of consumer health technologies may occur with even limited, and short-term use.
- User-centered design likely improves the utility, usability and usage of technology implementations; caregiver and veteran participation in the design and development of consumer health technologies should be solicited.
- Pre-implementation planning and budgets should assign resources to assist caregivers and veterans with access issues and ongoing technical support, and programs should assess the optimal levels of technical assistance and training required.
- Programs should assess how technologies can be tailored to the language and cultural needs of the caregiver and Veteran.
- Study whether formal online peer support groups exclusive to the VA have advantages over existing informal online interest groups.
- Caregivers and patients may seek immediately useful and relevant information online, such as skills improvement and assistance identifying community and financial resources. Future technology implementation interventions should explore their utility and methods for keeping information current.
- There is a need for more studies using mixed-methods and formative evaluation methods to help clarify effects and implementation strategies for these complex health technology interventions.

- There are several future research questions that may be of interest:
  - What are the optimal methods for implementing consumer health technologies in existing healthcare systems?
  - Does the use of consumer health technologies such as chat rooms, online peer support groups, and text messing with providers replace or complement face-to-face interactions?
  - How are consumer health technologies integrated into the day-to-day lives of caregivers?
  - How do caregiver demographics affect the user experience?
  - Are there differences between caregivers and Veterans in the user experience?
  - Develop tools to enhance caregiver-Veteran communication.
  - Studying the implementation of interventions within the VA using tools with broad reach, such as My HealtheVet.

REFERENCES

1. Jimison H, Gorman P, Woods S, et al. Barriers and Drivers of Health Information Technology Use for the Elderly, Chronically Ill, and Underserved. *AHRQ Publication No. 09-E004.* 2008;Evidence Report/Technology Assessment No. 175.

2. Gibbons MC, Wilson RF, Samal L, et al. Impact of Consumer Health Informatics Applications. *Agency for Healthcare Research and Quality. Evidence Report/Technology Assessment No. 188.* 2009;AHRQ Publication No. 09(10)-E019.

3. Nielsen J. *Designing Web Usability: The Practice of Simplicity.* Indianapolis: New Riders Publishing; 1999.

4. Brennan PF, Downs SM, Casper G. Project HealthDesign: Rethinking the power and potential of personal health records. *Journal of Biomedical Informatics.* 2010;43(5 Suppl):S3-5.

5. Houser A, Gibson MJ. Valuing the Invaluable: The Economic Value of Family Caregiving, 2008 Update. AARP Public Policy Institute, From Insight on the Issues 13, November, 2008. http://www.aarp.org/ppi (accessed 6/11/2012).

6. Fox S. Health Topics. Report of the Pew Internet & American Life Project, Feb 1, 2011, http://pewinternet.org/Reports/2011/HealthTopics.aspx, Accessed 6/11/2012.

7. Fox S, Jones S. The Social Life of Health Information. Report of the Pew Internet & American Life Project, May 12, 2011. http://pewinternet.org/Reports/2011/Social-Life-of-Health-Info.aspex, accessed 6/11/2012.

8. Zickuhr K, Smith A. Digital differences. Report of the Pew Research Center's Internet & American Life Project. April 13. 2012.

9. McInnes DK, Gifford AL, Kazis LE, Wagner TH. Disparities in health-related internet use by US veterans: results from a national survey. *Informatics in Primary Care.* 2010;18(1):59-68.

10. Anonymous. Consumer Health Informatics Taxonomy Delphi Study at Saint Louis University. https://slu.qualtrics.com/SE/?SID=SV_bqq7PCrC1Vo96GE. Accessed on 6/13. 2012. Accessed 6/13/2012.

11. Ahern DK, Woods SS, Lightowler MC, Finley SW, Houston TK. Promise of and Potential for Patient-Facing Technologies to Enable Meaningful Use. *Am J Prev Med.* 2011;40(5S2):S162-S172.

12. Anonymous. Best Care Together: Meeting Veterans Needs with Health Information Technology.2011.

13. Craig P, Dieppe P, MacIntyre S, Michie S, Nazareth I, Petticrew M. Developing and evaluating complex interventions: new guidance. Medical Research Council (MRC). Accessed June 7, 2012. http://www.mrc.ac.uk/complexinterventionsguidance. 2008.

14. Vehvilainen L, Zielstorff R, Gertman P, Tzeng M, Estey G. Alzheimer's Caregiver Internet Support System (ACISS): Evaluating the Feasibility and Effectiveness of Supporting Family Caregivers Virtually. Paper presented at: AMIA Annual Symposium Proceedings 2002.

15. Becker SA, Webbe F. Use of Handheld Technology by Older Adult Caregivers as Part of a Virtual Support Network. Paper presented at: Pervasive Health Conference and Workshops, 2006; Nov.-Dec. 2006, 2006.

16. Beauchamp N, Irvine AB, Seeley J, Johnson B. Worksite-based internet multimedia program for family caregivers of persons with dementia. *Gerontologist.* Dec 2005;45(6):793-801.

17. Chiu T, Lottridge D. Development and iterative refinement of an internet-based service for Chinese family caregivers of people with Alzheimer Disease. *AMIA Annu Symp Proc.* 2005:919.

18. Chiu T, Marziali E, Colantonio A, et al. Internet-based caregiver support for Chinese Canadians taking care of a family member with alzheimer disease and related dementia. *Can J Aging.* Dec 2009;28(4):323-336.

19. Bass DM, McClendon MJ, Brennan PF, McCarthy C. The buffering effect of a computer support network on caregiver strain. *Journal of Aging & Health.* Feb 1998;10(1):20-43.

20. Brennan PF, Moore SM, Smyth KA. The effects of a special computer network on caregivers of persons with Alzheimer's disease. *Nursing research.* May-Jun 1995;44(3):166-172.

21. Kuwahara N, Kuwabara K, Utsumi A, Yasuda K, Tetsutani N. Networked interaction therapy: relieving stress in memory-impaired people and their family members. *Conf Proc IEEE Eng Med Biol Soc.* 2004;5:3140-3143.

22. Hill-Kayser CE, Vachani C, Hampshire MK, Jacobs LA, Metz JM. An internet tool for creation of cancer survivorship care plans for survivors and health care providers: design, implementation, use and user satisfaction. *J Med Internet Res.* 2009;11(3):e39.

23. Namkoong K, Dubenske LL, Shaw BR, et al. Creating a Bond Between Caregivers Online: Effect on Caregivers' Coping Strategies. *J Health Commun.* Oct 17 2011.

24. Nolan MT, Hodgin MB, Olsen SJ, et al. Spiritual issues of family members in a pancreatic cancer chat room. *Oncol Nurs Forum.* Mar 2006;33(2):239-244.

25. Diefenbach MA, Butz BP. A multimedia interactive education system for prostate cancer patients: development and preliminary evaluation. *J Med Internet Res.* Jan 21 2004;6(1):e3.

26. Pierce LL, Steiner VL, Khuder SA, Govoni AL, Horn LJ. The effect of a Web-based stroke intervention on carers' well-being and survivors' use of healthcare services. *Disabil Rehabil.* 2009;31(20):1676-1684.

27. Steiner V, Pierce L, Drahuschak S, Nofziger E, Buchman D, Szirony T. Emotional support, physical help, and health of caregivers of stroke survivors. *J Neurosci Nurs.* Feb 2008;40(1):48-54.

28. Keaton L, Pierce LL, Steiner V, et al. An E-rehabilitation Team Helps Caregivers Deal with Stroke. *The Internet Journal of Allied Health Sciences and Practice.* 2004;2(4).

29. Pierce LL, Steiner V, Govoni AL, Hicks B, Cervantez Thompson TL, Friedemann ML. Internet-based support for rural caregivers of persons with stroke shows promise. *Rehabil Nurs.* Vol 29. 2004/05/22 ed2004:95-99, 103.

30. Pierce LL, Steiner V, Govoni AL, Hicks B, Cervantez Thompson TL, Friedemann M. Caregivers Dealing with Stroke Pull together and Feel Connected. *Journal of Neuroscience Nursing.* 2004;36(a).

31. Pierce LL, Steiner V, Govoni AL. In-home online support for caregivers of survivors of stroke: a feasibility study. *Comput Inform Nurs.* Jul-Aug 2002;20(4):157-164.

32. Stjernsward S, Ostman M. Illuminating user experience of a website for the relatives of persons with depression. *Int J Soc Psychiatry.* Jul 2011;57(4):375-386.

33. Glynn SM, Randolph ET, Garrick T, Lui A. A proof of concept trial of an online psychoeducational program for relatives of both veterans and civilians living with schizophrenia. *Psychiatr Rehabil J.* Spring 2010;33(4):278-287.

34. Rotondi AJ, Sinkule J, Spring M. An interactive Web-based intervention for persons with TBI and their families: use and evaluation by female significant others. *J Head Trauma Rehabil.* Mar-Apr 2005;20(2):173-185.

35. Rotondi AJ, Haas GL, Anderson CM, et al. A clinical trial to test the feasibility of a telehealth psychoeducational intervention for persons with schizophrenia and their families: intervention and 3-month findings. *Rehabilitation Psychology.* 2005;50(4):325-336.

36. Chiu T, Massimi M. A Digital Support Device Designed to Help Family Caregivers Coordinate, Communicate and Plan the Care of People with Brain Injury. *AMIA Symposium Proceedings.* 2006:884.

37. Huang F, Liu SC, Shih SM, et al. Reducing the anxiety of surgical patient's families access short message service. *AMIA Annu Symp Proc.* 2006:957.

38. Dew MA, Goycoolea JM, Harris RC, et al. An internet-based intervention to improve psychosocial outcomes in heart transplant recipients and family caregivers: development and evaluation. *J Heart Lung Transplant.* Jun 2004;23(6):745-758.

39. Chambers M, Connor SL. User-friendly technology to help family carers cope. *J Adv Nurs.* Dec 2002;40(5):568-577.

40. Magnusson L, Hanson E. Supporting frail older people and their family carers at home using information and communication technology: cost analysis. *J Adv Nurs.* Sep 2005;51(6):645-657.

41. Magnusson L. The impact of information and communication technology on family carers of older people and professionals in Sweden. *Ageing and Society.* 2005(25).

42. Finn J. An exploration of helping processes in an online self-help group focusing on issues of disability. *Health Soc Work.* 1999;24.

43. Fitzgerald SA, Macan Yadrich D, Werkowitch M, Piamjariyakul U, Smith CE. Creating patient and family education web sites: design and content of the home parenteral nutrition family caregivers web site. *Comput Inform Nurs.* Nov 2011;29(11):637-645.

44. Ossebaard HC, van Gemert-Pijnen JE, Sorbi MJ, Seydel ER. A study of a Dutch online decision aid for parents of children with ADHD. *J Telemed Telecare.* 2010;16(1):15-19.

45. Stinson J, McGrath P, Hodnett E, et al. Usability testing of an online self-management program for adolescents with juvenile idiopathic arthritis. *J Med Internet Res.* 2010;12(3):e30.

46. Krishna S, Francisco B, Boren SA, Balas EA. Evaluation of a Web-based Interactive Multimedia Pediatric Asthma Education Program. Paper presented at: AMIA Symposium Proceedings2000.

47. Krishna S, Francisco BD, Balas EA, et al. Internet-enabled interactive multimedia asthma education program: a randomized trial. *Pediatrics.* Mar 2003;111(3):503-510.

48. Bergmo TS, Wangberg SC, Schopf TR, Solvoll T. Web-based consultations for parents of children with atopic dermatitis: results of a randomized controlled trial. *Acta Paediatr.* Feb 2009;98(2):316-320.

49. Askins MA, Sahler OJ, Sherman SA, et al. Report from a multi-institutional randomized clinical trial examining computer-assisted problem-solving skills training for English- and Spanish-speaking mothers of children with newly diagnosed cancer. *J Pediatr Psychol.* Jun 2009;34(5):551-563.

50. Ewing LJ, Long K, Rotondi A, Howe C, Bill L, Marsland AL. Brief report: A pilot study of a web-based resource for families of children with cancer. *J Pediatr Psychol.* Jun 2009;34(5):523-529.

51. Han HR, Belcher AE. Computer-mediated support group use among parents of children with cancer--an exploratory study. *Comput Nurs.* Jan-Feb 2001;19(1):27-33.

52. Lewis D, Cooper J, Gunawardena S. Caring Connection: Internet resources for family caregivers of children with cancer. *AMIA Annu Symp Proc.* 2006:1007.

53. Gulmans J, Vollenbroek-Hutten MM, Visser JJ, Nijeweme-d'Hollosy WO, van Gemert-Pijnen JE, van Harten WH. A web-based communication system for integrated care in cerebral palsy: design features, technical feasibility and usability. *J Telemed Telecare.* 2010;16(7):389-393.

54. Britto MT, Jimison HB, Munafo JK, Wissman J, Rogers ML, Hersh W. Usability testing finds problems for novice users of pediatric portals. *J Am Med Inform Assoc.* Sep-Oct 2009;16(5):660-669.

55. Nelson TM, Berg JH, Bell JF, Leggott PJ, Seminario AL. Assessing the effectiveness of text messages as appointment reminders in a pediatric dental setting. *J Am Dent Assoc.* Apr 2011;142(4):397-405.

56. Demaso DR, Marcus NE, Kinnamon C, Gonzalez-Heydrich J. Depression experience journal: a computer-based intervention for families facing childhood depression. *J Am Acad Child Adolesc Psychiatry.* Feb 2006;45(2):158-165.

57. Keshavjee K, Lawson ML, Malloy M, Hubbard S, Grass M. Technology failure analysis: understanding why a diabetes management tool developed for a Personal Digital Assistant (PDA) didn't work in a randomized controlled trial. *AMIA Annu Symp Proc.* 2003:889.

58. Nordfeldt S, Hanberger L, Bertero C. Patient and parent views on a Web 2.0 Diabetes Portal--the management tool, the generator, and the gatekeeper: qualitative study. *J Med Internet Res.* 2010;12(2):e17.

59. Stockwell MS, Kharbanda EO, Martinez RA, et al. Effect of a text messaging intervention on influenza vaccination in an urban, low-income pediatric and adolescent population: a randomized controlled trial. *JAMA.* April 25 2012;307(16):1702-1708.

60. Miloh T, Annunziato R, Arnon R, et al. Improved adherence and outcomes for pediatric liver transplant recipients by using text messaging. *Pediatrics.* Nov 2009;124(5):e844-850.

61. Safran C, Pompilio-Weitzner G, Emery KD, Hampers L. A Medicaid eHealth program: an analysis of benefits to users and nonusers. *AMIA Annu Symp Proc.* 2005:659-663.

62. Goldman RD, Antoon R, Tait G, Zimmer D, Viegas A, Mounstephen B. Culture results via the internet: a novel way for communication after an emergency department visit. *J Pediatr.* Aug 2005;147(2):221-226.

63. Mindell JA, Du Mond CE, Sadeh A, Telofski LS, Kulkarni N, Gunn E. Efficacy of an internet-based intervention for infant and toddler sleep disturbances. *Sleep.* Apr 2011;34(4):451-458.

64. Wade SL, Carey J, Wolfe CR. An online family intervention to reduce parental distress following pediatric brain injury. *J Consult Clin Psychol.* Jun 2006;74(3):445-454.

65. Carey JC, Wade SL, Wolfe CR. Lessons learned: the effect of prior technology use on Web-based interventions. *Cyberpsychol Behav.* Apr 2008;11(2):188-195.

66. Wade SL, Wolfe CR, Pestian JP. A web-based family problem-solving intervention for families of children with traumatic brain injury. *Behav Res Methods Instrum Comput.* May 2004;36(2):261-269.

67. Wade SL, Walz NC, Carey JC, Williams KM. Preliminary efficacy of a Web-based family problem-solving treatment program for adolescents with traumatic brain injury. *J Head Trauma Rehabil.* Nov-Dec 2008;23(6):369-377.

68. Wade SL, Walz NC, Carey JC, Williams KM. Brief report: Description of feasibility and satisfaction findings from an innovative online family problem-solving intervention for adolescents following traumatic brain injury. *J Pediatr Psychol.* Jun 2009;34(5):517-522.

69. Marsac ML, Kassam-Adams N, Hildenbrand AK, Kohser KL, Winston FK. After the injury: initial evaluation of a web-based intervention for parents of injured children. *Health Educ Res.* Feb 2011;26(1):1-12.

70. *Impact of a Patient Portal to Improve Quality of Care in an Autism Clinic* 2011.

71. Glueckauf RL, Ketterson TU, Loomis JS, Dages P. Online support and education for dementia caregivers: overview, utilization, and initial program evaluation. *Telemed J E Health.* Summer 2004;10(2):223-232.

72. Becker SA, Webbe F. The Potential of Hand-held Assistive Technology to Improve Safety for Elder Adults Aging in Place. *In K. Henriksen, J. B. Battles, M. A. Keyes, and D. I. Lewin (Eds.), Advances in Patient Safety: New Directions and Alternative Approaches, Bethesda, MD: Agency for Healthcare Research and Quality (AHRQ), 107-119.* 2008.

73. Magnusson L. A literature review study of Information and Communication Technology as a support for frail older people living at home and their family carers. *Technology and Disability.* 2004;16:223-235. 214, 221-213.

74. Magnusson L, Hanson E. *Support "online" for older people and their family carers -- the EU project ACTION... Assisting Carers using Telematics Interventions to meet Older person's Needs.* Geneva, Switzerland: International Council of Nurses; 2001.

75. Usability Professionals' Association. What is user-centered design? http://www.usabilityprofessionals.org/usability_resources/about_usability/what_is_ucd.html, accessed June 14, 2012.

76. Smith A. 17% of cell phone owners do most of their online browsing on their phone, rather than a computer or other device. *Pew Research Center's Internet & American Life Project.* 2012;http://pewinternet.org/Reports/2012/Cell-Internet-Use-2012.aspx.

77. U.S. Department of Health & Human Services. Usability.gov - Your guide for developing usable & useful Web sites. http://www.usability.gov/ Accessed October 25, 2012.

78. McLean S, Chandler D, Nurmatov U, et al. Telehealthcare for Asthma: A Cochrane Review. *CMAJ.* 2011;183(11):E733-742.

79. McLean S, Nurmatov U, Liu JL, Pagliari C, Car J, Sheikh A. Telehealthcare for Chronic Obstructive Pulmonary Disease. *Cochrane Database of Systematic Reviews.* 2011(7).

80. Farmer A, Gibson OJ, Tarassenko L, Neil A. A Systematic Review of Telemedicine Interventions to Support Blood Glucose Self-monitoring in Diabetes. *Diabet Med.* 2005;22(10):1372-1378.

81. Hersh WR, Hickam DH, Severance SM, Dana TL, Krages KP, Helfand M. Telemedicine for the Medicare Population: Update. *Evid Rep Technol Assess (Full Rep).* 2006(131):1-41.

82. Greist JH, Osgood-Hynes DJ, Baer L, Marks IM. Technology-Based Advances in the Management of Depression: Focus on the COPE(TM) Program. *Disease Management & Health Outcomes.* 2000;7(4):193-200(198).

83. McDaniel AM, Benson PL, Roesener GH, Martindale J. An integrated computer-based system to support nicotine dependence treatment in primary care. *Nicotine & Tobacco Research.* Apr 2005;7 Suppl 1:S57-66.

84. Forster AJ, van Walraven C. Using an interactive voice response system to improve patient safety following hospital discharge. *J Eval Clin Pract.* Jun 2007;13(3):346-351.

85. Piette JD. Interactive voice response systems in the diagnosis and management of chronic disease. *Am J Manag Care.* Jul 2000;6(7):817-827.

86. Piette JD, Datwani H, Gaudioso S, et al. Hypertension management using mobile technology and home blood pressure monitoring: results of a randomized trial in two low/middle-income countries. *Telemedicine Journal & E-Health.* Oct 2012;18(8):613-620.

87. Handley MA, Shumway M, Schillinger D. Cost-effectiveness of automated telephone self-management support with nurse care management among patients with diabetes. *Ann Fam Med.* Nov-Dec 2008;6(6):512-518.

APPENDIX A. SEARCH STRATEGY

Search conducted in MEDLINE® via PubMed® on 12/9/2011

Concept	Search#	Search String	Citations
Non-Professional caregivers	#60	(("Family"[Mesh]) OR "Caregivers"[Mesh]) OR "Home Nursing"[Mesh]	220979
	#77	(((caregiv*[Title/Abstract]) OR "care giving"[Title/Abstract]) OR "care giver"[Title/Abstract]) OR care givers[Title/Abstract]	28393
	#78	(#77) OR #60	235910
Mobile apps	#80	(("Computers, Handheld"[Mesh]) OR "Cellular Phone"[Mesh]) OR "wireless technology"[Mesh]	4152
	#81	iPad OR handheld OR interactive OR mobile computing OR smart phone* OR mobile phone* OR mobile technolog* OR m-health OR internet based OR personal digital assistant* OR online OR sms OR iphone OR android OR text messag* OR tablet computer OR informatics application OR app	100411
	#82	(#81) OR #80	101517
Union of concepts	#83	(#82) AND #78	2147

Search for specialized databases and grey literature conducted 12/9/2011 and 4/30/2012

Specialized Databases and Grey literature sources searched		
Database	Search	Hits
AMIA Proceedings http://proceedings.amia.org Searched 12/9/2011	"caregiv*"	268
IEEE Xplore http://ieeexplore.ieee.org Searched 12/9/2011	"caregiv*"	266
Healthcare Information & management Systems (HiMSS) conferences and website http://www.himss.org/ASP/index.asp Searched 4/30/2012	"caregiver" OR "caregiving"	2
Med 2.0 (abstracts from 2008 – 2012) http://www.medicine20congress.com/ocs/index.php/med/med2012 Searched 4/30/2012	"caregiver" OR "caregiving"	2
Health 2.0 (abstracts from 2007 – 2011) http://www.health2con.com/conferences/ Searched 4/30/2012	"caregiver" OR "caregiving"	No results

APPENDIX B. INCLUSION/EXCLUSION CRITERIA

1. Is the full text of the article in English?
   Yes .... Proceed to #2
   No .... Code **X1**. STOP

2. Is the article a primary study that presents findings based on original data collection; or a systematic review of primary studies?
   Yes .... Proceed to #3
   No .... Code **X2**. Go to #6

3. Does the article evaluate the effectiveness of a targeted consumer health information technology (CHIT) intervention listed below in the PICOTS?
   Yes .... Proceed to #4
   No .... Code **X3**. Go to #5

4. Does the study population include non-professional, human/non-robot caregivers of patients with chronic illness or disability, or are caregiver-centered outcomes reported as a primary outcome?
   Yes, adult patients .... Code **I3/A**. STOP
   Yes, child patients .... Code **I3/C**. STOP
   No .... Code **X4**. Go to #6

5. Is the article a primary study or systematic review evaluating the effects of telephony, interactive voice response, or telehealth interventions?
   Yes .... Code **I5**. STOP
   No .... Code **X5**. Go to #6

6. Is the article possibly useful for background/discussion? .... Code **B**. STOP

PICOTS:

Population: Non-professional, non-robot caregivers of adult patients with chronic illnesses, and/or parents of children with healthcare needs.

Intervention: Self-directed mobile applications for use on smart phones, personal digital assistants (PDAs) and tablet computers, including: interactive or individually tailored web-based interventions, decision aids, and risk assessment software; chat and online support groups; secure messaging; or other portable or home-based interactive information tools whose purpose is to facilitate communication, coordination, or tailored education in order to support the emotional, spiritual, organizational, management, and healthcare needs of non-professional caregivers of patients with chronic illnesses or health risk factors. Non-interactive educational media (e.g., E-pamphlet) that provide information only are excluded.

We excluded studies focused on telephony, interactive-voice-response, synchronous telehealth interventions, and fixed home-monitoring technologies such as smart-homes, vitals-monitoring, GPS and other location-monitoring, and monitoring for patient falls.

Control: Usual care (use of paper forms and educational materials, in-person visits).

Outcomes:

1) *Caregiver-centered outcomes:* caregiver satisfaction, caregiver burnout, caregiver access, caregiver quality of life scores, caregiver depression/anxiety scores.

2) *Patient-centered outcomes:* patient satisfaction, patient activation, functional status, quality of life; quality of patient-caregiver relationship.

3) *Process measures:* clinician satisfaction; caregiver perceptions of mobile technologies; usage, usability, and barriers to usage of technologies/tools/applications; communication with healthcare providers.

4) *Utilization outcomes:* hospitalizations, ER visits, outpatient/PCP visits.

Timing: No restrictions.

Setting: Outpatient (home, assisted living, adult foster care), excluding skilled nursing facilities.

www.ingramcontent.com/pod-product-compliance
Lightning Source LLC
Chambersburg PA
CBHW082031190526
45166CB00017B/2940